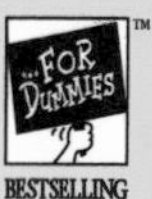

BESTSELLING BOOK SERIES

Osteoporosis For

Best Dietary Cal

Fortified milk	
Canned sardines	
Almonds	
Calcium-fortified orange juice	300 mg per cup
Yogurt, low fat, plain	300 mg per cup
Figs, dried	270 mg in 10 figs
Turnip greens	250 mg per cup, cooked from frozen
Spinach	250 mg per cup, cooked from raw and drained
Cheese, hard	240 mg per ounce
Oysters, raw	225 milligram per cup
Cheese pizza	220 mg in one slice
Quiche Lorraine	210 mg per slice
Cream of chicken soup	180 mg in a cup made with milk
Salmon, canned, with bones	180 mg per 3 ounces
Oatmeal, instant, fortified	160 mg per packet
Peanuts	125 mg per cup
Cottage cheese	120 mg per cup
Beans, white	100 mg per cup
Yogurt, frozen	100 mg per half cup
Cheese enchilada	97 mg in one enchilada

Dietary Sources of Vitamin D

Salmon, canned	360 IU per 3 ounces
Milk	100 IU per cup
Margarine, fortified	60 IU per 2 teaspoons
Cereals, fortified	40 to 80 IU per serving
Egg, 1 whole	20 IU

For Dummies: Bestselling Book Series for Beginners

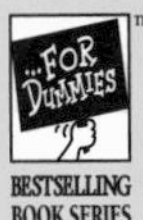

Osteoporosis For Dummies®

Cheat Sheet

Preventing Falls: A Checklist of Things to Watch Out For

- **Alcohol:** Be sure to keep your alcoholic beverage intake to a minimum, to prevent you from losing your balance.
- **Bathrooms:** Have grab bars and nonslip bathmats or tape installed in your tub and shower.
- **Floors:** Reduce clutter and secure or remove all loose wires, cords, and throw rugs. Make sure all your rugs are anchored and have no wrinkles or bumps.
- **Kitchen:** Always clean spills immediately, especially from the floor, and install nonskid rubber mats near the sink, stove, and refrigerator.
- **Lighting:** Make sure all your halls, stairways, and entrances are well lit. If you get up in the middle of the night, be sure to turn your lights on so you can easily see where you're going. Install a night light in your bathroom.
- **Medications:** Ask your doctor whether any of your medications might cause dizziness and make you fall.
- **Shoes:** Be sure to always wear sturdy, rubber-soled shoes to reduce slippage.
- **Stairs:** Make sure all the treads, rails, and rugs in your house are secure.

What You Can Do to Decrease the Effects of Osteoporosis

Meet your Calcium requirement:	1,200 to 1,500 mg daily
Meet your Vitamin D requirement:	600 to 800 IU daily

Weight-bearing exercise at least three times a week

Quit smoking

Limit alcohol to one to two drinks per day

Have a DXA scan done

For Dummies: Bestselling Book Series for Beginners

Osteoporosis FOR DUMMIES®

by Carolyn Riester O'Connor, MD

Sharon Perkins, RN

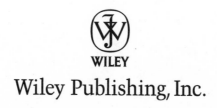

Wiley Publishing, Inc.

Osteoporosis For Dummies®

Published by
Wiley Publishing, Inc.
111 River St.
Hoboken, NJ 07030-5774
www.wiley.com

Published by Wiley Publishing, Inc., Indianapolis, Indiana

Published simultaneously in Canada

Library of Congress Control Number: 2005923787

ISBN-13: 978-0-7645-7621-8

ISBN-10: 0-7645-7621-6

Manufactured in the United States of America

10 9 8 7 6 5 4 3 2 1

1B/RW/QW/QV/IN

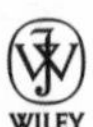

About the Authors

Carolyn O'Connor graduated *cum laude* from Yale College with a bachelor of science degree in chemistry. She then traveled to Manhattan to attend Columbia College of Physicians and Surgeons. After medical school, she did her postgraduate training in internal medicine at The New York Hospital – Cornell Medical School. Her fellowship training in rheumatology was at Boston University Medical Center. Currently, she is chief of rheumatology and associate professor of medicine at Drexel University College of Medicine in Philadelphia. One of her major interests is metabolic bone disease. Her division of rheumatology runs the bone density program at Drexel.

She has two children; one has majored in philosophy and the other is studying mechanical engineering. Her outside interests include growing roses and struggling with the *New York Times* Crossword.

Sharon Perkins has been a registered nurse for almost 20 years, and currently works for a group of retinal doctors. Since she started treating an older population with macular degeneration, she sees way more osteoporosis than she wishes she did. She has five children and two daughters-in-law, two grandchildren, and a husband who recently retired from 20-plus years of flying airplanes and is currently hanging around the house.

Dedications

I dedicate this book to my many patients who trust in my advice. Truly, from listening to them and caring for them, I have learned more about osteoporosis than from reading any textbook.

Carolyn R. O'Connor, MD

For my granddaughter Emma, in hopes that osteoporosis will be fully preventable in her future.

Sharon Perkins

Author Acknowledgments

Many thanks to the following people:

* Antonio J Reginato, MD (in memoriam) friend and mentor, who taught me about metabolic bone disease and showed me my first case of osteomalacia 20 years ago
* Gerald F. Falasca, MD, who taught me how to read my first bone density reading
* Norman A. Johanson, MD, Chief of Orthopedic Surgery, Drexel University College of Medicine, who contributed invaluable comments to Chapter 13
* Susan Ott, MD, who supplied pathologic slides of bone disorders

Carolyn R. O'Connor, MD

One of my earliest memories is of my great grandmother, who my younger sister called "the grandma with the broken arm." I'd just met my family history of osteoporosis, although I didn't know it at the time.

Years down the road, my children remembered *their* great grandmother, daughter of my great grandma, who had fallen and broken her hip. Pictures show the inches she lost as she aged as evidence of vertebral compression fractures.

Osteoporosis runs in my family, but we never really put a name to it or did much about it. But because of the problems my relatives had, I was always aware of aging as being dangerous for your bones, and for that, I thank them.

I also have to thank my sister, Sue, for telling me I'd hate writing a book on osteoporosis, because "bones are boring." She knows I love a challenge.

Thanks to all the rest of my family and my friends for occasionally remembering that I was writing a book and asking me how it was going. Sometimes I needed a chance to vent!

For all the people behind the scenes at Wiley Publishing, especially Kathy Cox, who never loses faith in me, thank you.

Dr. O'Connor and I both thank our acquisitions editor, Mikal Belicove, for the chance to write this book, as well as our marvelous project editor, Natalie Harris, copy editor, Chad Sievers, and technical editor, Deborah Kado. And once again, Kathryn Born has done a wonderful job on illustrations.

Sharon Perkins

Publisher's Acknowledgments

We're proud of this book; please send us your comments through our Dummies online registration form located at www.dummies.com/register/.

Some of the people who helped bring this book to market include the following:

Acquisitions, Editorial, and Media Development

Project Editor: Natalie Faye Harris

Acquisitions Editor: Mikal E. Belicove

Copy Editor: Chad Sievers

General Reviewer: Deborah Kado, MD, MS

Senior Permissions Editor: Carmen Krikorian

Editorial Manager: Michelle Hacker

Editorial Assistants: Courtney Allen, Melissa Bennett

Cover Photos: Steve Bly/Getty Images/Stone

Illustrations: Kathryn Born

Cartoons: Rich Tennant, www.the5thwave.com

Composition

Project Coordinator: Nancee Reeves

Layout and Graphics: Carl Byers, Andrea Dahl, Lauren Goddard, Stephanie D. Jumper, Mary Gillot Virgin

Proofreaders: Leeann Harney, Carl William Pierce, Dwight Ramsey, TECHBOOKS Production Services

Indexer: TECHBOOKS Production Services

Publishing and Editorial for Consumer Dummies

Diane Graves Steele, Vice President and Publisher, Consumer Dummies

Joyce Pepple, Acquisitions Director, Consumer Dummies

Kristin A. Cocks, Product Development Director, Consumer Dummies

Michael Spring, Vice President and Publisher, Travel

Kelly Regan, Editorial Director, Travel

Publishing for Technology Dummies

Andy Cummings, Vice President and Publisher, Dummies Technology/General User

Composition Services

Gerry Fahey, Vice President of Production Services

Debbie Stailey, Director of Composition Services

Contents at a Glance

Introduction ***1***

Part I: Understanding Your Bones ***7***

Chapter 1: Boning Up on Osteoporosis 9
Chapter 2: Loving the Living Tissue Called Bone 19
Chapter 3: Breaking Down the Risk Factors 33
Chapter 4: Men and Kids Get Osteoporosis, Too 53

Part II: Keeping Your Bones Healthy ***69***

Chapter 5: Eating Right for Good Bones 71
Chapter 6: Exercising for Strong Bones 87

Part III: Diagnosing and Treating Osteoporosis ***105***

Chapter 7: Facing the Consequences of Bones Gone Bad 107
Chapter 8: Finding (and Paying For) a Doctor to Treat Osteoporosis 119
Chapter 9: Testing Your Bones 133
Chapter 10: Taking Prescription Drugs for Osteoporosis 145
Chapter 11: Keeping Bones Strong with Over-the-Counter Supplements 161
Chapter 12: Managing Pain from Osteoporosis 177
Chapter 13: Recovering from a Fracture When You Have Osteoporosis 193
Chapter 14: Focusing on the Future of Osteoporosis 213

Part IV: The Part of Tens ***225***

Chapter 15: Ten Surprising Sources of Calcium 227
Chapter 16: Ten Things You Need to Know about Bones 231
Chapter 17: Ten Resources for Finding Out More about Osteoporosis 237
Chapter 18: Top Ten Questions Dr. O'Connor's Patients Ask about Osteoporosis 243
Chapter 19: Ten (Or So) Parenting Tips to Build Strong Bones 247

Appendix: Reviewing Osteoporosis Programs State by State ***251***

Glossary ***263***

Index..***271***

Table of Contents

Introduction 1

About This Book 2
Conventions Used in This Book 2
What You're Not to Read 3
Foolish Assumptions 3
How This Book Is Organized 4
Part I: Understanding Your Bones 4
Part II: Keeping Bones Healthy 4
Part III: Diagnosing and Treating Osteoporosis 4
Part IV: The Part of Tens 4
Icons Used in This Book 5
Where to Go from Here 5

Part I: Understanding Your Bones 7

Chapter 1: Boning Up on Osteoporosis 9

Defining Osteoporosis 9
Who, Me? How Osteoporosis May Affect You 10
Looking more closely at the numbers:
How serious is osteoporosis? 11
Defeating fragility fractures before they occur 12
Uncovering the relationship between
aging and osteoporosis 13
Why Early Diagnosis Is So Important 13
Improving Your Peak Bone Density —
And Your Children's 14
Evaluating Osteoporosis Therapy 16
Terminology 101: Keeping Your "Osteos" Straight 16
Osteoarthritis: It hurts, but it's not osteoporosis 16
Osteomalacia: So why exactly
did that bone break? 17
Osteopenia warning: Falling bone density ahead! 18

Chapter 2: Loving the Living Tissue Called Bone 19

Understanding Your Living Skeleton 19
Meeting Your Bones 21
Looking at the different types of bones 22
Examining the innards and outards of your bones ...22
Modeling and Remodeling 24

Building Up and Breaking Down: Your Bones Day by Day ..25
Blasts, clasts, and cytes (oh my) 25
Fine-tuning your bones with hormones 26
Orchestrating bone growth with minerals 28
Your Bones from Birth to Infinity: More Stuff to Know 29

Chapter 3: Breaking Down the Risk Factors 33

Assessing Your Risk Factors: Which Women Get Osteoporosis? 34
I am woman, see me shrink 34
Aging is such sweet sorrow 35
Blaming it on the family 35
Weighty issues 36
Starting and stopping menstrual periods 40
Focusing on Lifestyle Factors 40
Smoking and osteoporosis 40
How alcohol affects your bones 41
Watching what you eat 42
Recognizing Medications That Cause Bone Loss 43
Why corticosteroids can thin bones 44
Avoiding excess thyroid medication 45
Taking medications to prevent seizures 46
Other drugs associated with developing osteoporosis 46
How Gastrointestinal Problems Can Affect Your Bones 47
Inflammatory bowel disease 47
Bone loss after stomach surgery 48
Celiac disease and bone loss 48
Noting Other Diseases Associated with Osteoporosis 48
Reducing the Risks of Getting Osteoporosis 50

Chapter 4: Men and Kids Get Osteoporosis, Too 53

Taking a Closer Look at Who Else Gets Osteoporosis 53
Focusing on Osteoporosis in Men 54
Seeking answers in the "Mr. OS" study 55
Treating men with osteoporosis 57
Prostate cancer and osteoporosis 58
Focusing on prevention and treatment 59
Why Too Thin Is Bad for Bones — Especially in Teens 60
Dieting and bone loss 60
The female athlete triad 62
Yes, Little Kids Can Have Osteoporosis 63
Rickets: A real risk for bone loss 63
Osteogenesis imperfecta (OI) 64
Corticosteroids and osteoporosis in children 66

Part II: Keeping Your Bones Healthy 69

Chapter 5: Eating Right for Good Bones **71**

Getting Enough Calcium in Your Diet 72
  Living with lactose intolerance 76
  "Eat your leafy greens!" 78
  Reading the labels: How much calcium is in it? 79
Examining the Critical Role of Vitamin D 80
Nutrients You Probably Never Think About 81
Setting Down the Saltshaker 82
High Protein or Low Protein? 82
Assessing Alcohol in Your Diet 83
Decreasing Caffeine: Does it Matter? 84
Looking At How Your Weight Affects Your Bones 85

Chapter 6: Exercising for Strong Bones **87**

Starting While You're Still Young 88
Moving Your Bones to Build More Bone 89
  Understanding why exercise strengthens bone 89
  Utilizing weight-bearing exercise and resistance training 89
Developing an Exercise Plan 90
  Setting an exercise schedule 91
  Finding time in your life for exercise 92
Avoiding Injury While Exercising 92
Getting Down to the Nitty-Gritty: Choosing an Exercise Routine 93
  Biceps curls with dumbbells 95
  Triceps kickback 96
  Overhead press 98
  Knee extensors 99
  Hip extensors 100
  Hip flexors 101
  Leg lifts 103

Part III: Diagnosing and Treating Osteoporosis 105

Chapter 7: Facing the Consequences of Bones Gone Bad **107**

Aging and Your Bones 107
Facing Fragility Fractures 108

Breaking Bones – Different Types of Fractures 109
Falling on outstretched arms 109
"I broke my hip! Or was it my femur?" 111
Falling and hip fractures 112
Developing a dowager's hump 114

Chapter 8: Finding (and Paying For) a Doctor to Treat Osteoporosis 119

I Looked in the Phonebook, But I Couldn't Find Any Bone-ologists 119
Seeing your family doctor 120
Choosing a specialist 120
Taking extra courses in bone: Metabolic bone specialists 121
Preparing to Meet the Doctor 122
Getting ready for your first appointment 123
Making sure you've found Dr. Right 124
Team Tactics: Setting Up a Care Plan with Your Doctor 124
Being honest with your doctor 126
Being honest with yourself 127
Keeping in touch after your visit 127
Getting the Most Out of Your Insurance Plan 128
Eeny meeny miney moe — did I choose an HMO? 129
Going out of network 131
Getting your drugs covered 131

Chapter 9: Testing Your Bones 133

What's Bone Density Testing, Anyway? 134
Deciding When to Have a Bone Density Test 134
DXA, SXA, PDXA, and More — Understanding This Alphabet Soup 136
Deciphering DXA 136
Settling for SXA 137
Pondering PDXA 138
Looking at the RA 138
Questioning pQCT 138
Testing Bones in Other Ways 138
Ultrasound tests 139
Blood and urine tests 139
Interpreting the Results of Your DXA 139
Knowing your T-score 140
Catching the Z's 141
Interpreting all these numbers 142
Knowing How Often You Need a Bone Density Test 143

Chapter 10: Taking Prescription Drugs for Osteoporosis 145

Sorting Out the Different Types of Drug Treatment 145
Looking at Bisphosphonates for Building Up Bone 147
Using alendronate, ibandronate, and risedronate ...147
Deciding when to treat with bisphosphonates 148
Who shouldn't take bisphosphonates? 149
Taking bisphosphonates correctly 149
The Estrogen Replacement Controversy 150
Taking estrogen correctly 151
Living with side effects of estrogen 153
Trying "designer estrogens" (Evista) 154
Calcitonin: An Old Medication Standby 155
Building Bone with Teripeptides 156
When to consider prevention 156
Deciding on testosterone replacement therapy.......157
Exploring New Directions in Medication 158
Administering bisphosphonates in a new manner 158
Combining drug therapies 159
Using ultra low-dose estrogen 159
Strontium 159
Tibolone (Livial) 160

Chapter 11: Keeping Bones Strong with Over-the-Counter Supplements 161

Why Vitamin D Is a Major Player 162
Checking your vitamin D levels 164
Drugs that interfere with vitamin D absorption 164
Correlating vitamin D deficiency and hip fractures 165
Reducing falls with vitamin D 165
Taking in too much vitamin D 165
Overdoing Vitamin A 166
Confronting the Cacophony of Calcium Supplements 167
Reading the labels for elemental calcium 168
Ingesting your daily calcium 169
Calcium interactions 170
Making sure your calcium dissolves 171
Getting the lead out 172
Combining calcium and other vitamins and minerals 173
Antacids for your bones? 174
Taking calcium when you have other medical conditions 175

Chapter 12: Managing Pain from Osteoporosis 177

Recognizing the Real Pain of Osteoporosis 178
"Oh, My Aching Back!" 179
Treating Acute Pain from a Fracture 180
- Narcotic medications for short-term pain 180
- OTC analgesics or NSAIDs? 181
- Non-narcotic prescription pain medications 184

Treating Chronic Pain: What to Do When Pain Goes On and On 185
- When pain medication makes you woozy 185
- Taking more than one medication 186
- Keeping an eye on addiction 186

Dealing with Pain without Medication 187
- Heating it up or cooling it down 187
- Using physical therapy 188
- Exercising to get rid of pain 188
- Exploring TENS units 189
- Trying acupuncture for chronic pain 189
- Massaging away the pain 190
- Bracing yourself, internally and externally 190
- Coping with pain psychologically 190
- Seeing a pain management guru 191

Chapter 13: Recovering from a Fracture When You Have Osteoporosis 193

Checking for Osteoporosis after a Fracture 194
Preventing Falls 194
Recognizing Breaks and What's Most Likely to Break 196
- Handling hip fractures 197
- Comprehending vertebral compression fractures 206
- With a snap of your wrist — a Colles' fracture 210
- Other kinds of fractures 211

How Long Does Bone Take to Heal? 211
Reducing the Chance of Another Fracture 212

Chapter 14: Focusing on the Future of Osteoporosis 213

Improving Osteoporosis Prevention 213
- How do doctors encourage patients to change habits? 214
- How are healthcare providers educated? 215
- Needing more research in prevention 216

Looking at Future Technologies for Your Bones 217
- Better diagnosing for fragile bone 217
- Understanding how your genes lead to osteoporosis 218

Finding Future Medications 218
New ways of giving bisphosphonates 219
Developing new drug compounds by studying bone biology 220
Repairing Collapsed Vertebrae: A New Surgical Treatment 220
Fighting Osteoporosis on an International Level 221
Battling Osteoporosis in the United States 222
Ongoing Research Regarding Osteoporosis 223

Part IV: The Part of Tens 225

Chapter 15: Ten Surprising Sources of Calcium 227

Drinking Mineral Water 227
Going Beyond Leafy Green Veggies 228
Munching on Nuts and Seeds 228
Eating Tacos for Dinner 229
Sending Out for Pizza 229
Taking One Latte to Go! 229
Chugging a Little OJ Today 229
Adding a Little Molasses 230
Indulging on Chocolate Cake 230
Powdering with a Different Twist 230

Chapter 16: Ten Things You Need to Know about Bones 231

Broken Bones Hurt! 231
Broken Bones Can Make You Sick — or Worse 232
Increasing Calcium Certainly Helps Decrease Fractures ..232
Milk Is Really Important to Bone 232
You Don't Get a Second Chance at Building Bone 233
Today's Bad Habits Lead to Tomorrow's Bone Loss 233
Getting Shorter Is No Fun at All 233
Your Bones Are a Storehouse of Necessary Minerals 234
Broken Bones Cost Society a Ton of Money 234
Bones Turn Over All the Time 235

Chapter 17: Ten Resources for Finding Out More about Osteoporosis 237

Staying Up-to-Date with the NOF 237
Relying on the NIH 238
Utilizing Expert Medical Facilities 239
Joining a Support Group 239
Chatting Online about Osteoporosis 239
Reading Books 240
Watching Videos 240
Talking with Your Doctor about Osteoporosis 241

Visiting Your Favorite Physical Therapist 241
Going Online for the Latest Information 241

Chapter 18: Top Ten Questions Dr. O'Connor's Patients Ask about Osteoporosis 243

What's the Best Type of Calcium for Me? 243
How Much Calcium Do I Need Each Day? 244
I Drink Plenty of Milk. Isn't That Enough Calcium for My Bones? 244
What Exercises Are Best for Preventing Osteoporosis? 244
What's the Difference between Osteoporosis and Osteoarthritis? 244
My Back Hurts. Is That My Osteoporosis? 245
What Else Can I Do to Improve Bone Strength? 245
My Family Doc Recommended a Bone Density Study. How Is It Done? 245
Which Is Better, Alendronate or Risedronate? 246
I've Had a Curved Spine Since My Teenage Years. Do I Have Osteoporosis? 246

Chapter 19: Ten (Or So) Parenting Tips to Build Strong Bones 247

The More You Exercise, the Stronger Your Bones Will Be 247
Drinking Milk Daily Builds Big Benefits for Bones 248
Shopping Wisely Is Worth the Extra Time 248
Don't Let Lactose Intolerance Rob Your Child of Calcium 248
Avoid Carbonated Beverages 249
Watch for Signs of Anorexia 249
Know Your Family History 249
Set an Example about Eating Healthy 250
Help Your Teen Avoid Cigarettes and Alcohol 250

Appendix: Reviewing Osteoporosis Programs State by State 251

Alabama 251
Alaska 251
Arizona 252
Arkansas 252
California 252
Colorado 252
Connecticut 253
Delaware 253

District of Columbia 253
Florida 253
Georgia 254
Hawaii 254
Idaho 254
Illinois 254
Indiana 254
Iowa 255
Kansas 255
Kentucky 255
Louisiana 255
Maine 255
Maryland 255
Massachusetts 256
Michigan 256
Minnesota 256
Mississippi 256
Missouri 256
Montana 257
Nebraska 257
Nevada 257
New Hampshire 257
New Jersey 257
New Mexico 258
New York 258
North Carolina 258
North Dakota 258
Ohio 258
Oklahoma 258
Oregon 259
Pennsylvania 259
Rhode Island 259
South Carolina 259
South Dakota 260
Tennessee 260
Texas 260
Utah 260
Vermont 260
Virginia 260
Washington 261
West Virginia 261
Wisconsin 261
Wyoming 261

Glossary 263

Index 271

Introduction

You may think you know enough about osteoporosis without reading a whole book on it. Take calcium, try not to fall down the basement steps, be prepared to shrink three or four inches as you get older, and so on, right? What else is there to know? Plenty, as we hope you'll agree after reading this book. The unfortunate fact is that although nobody wants to have osteoporosis, not enough people take steps to decrease their chances of developing it.

Considering that your odds of developing osteoporosis in the United States today are around 40 percent if you're female and 10 percent if you're male, many people are leaving the fate of their bones to chance.

One of our goals in writing this book is to keep you from developing osteoporosis. However, if you already have osteoporosis, our goal is to minimize the damage it does to your bones, through medication, healthy eating, and exercise.

If you've already fallen and broken bones, we want to help you avoid another fall. If you have children or grandchildren, we hope that you'll nag them into taking steps to avoid falling into osteoporosis themselves. We want to help you have healthy bones. We also want you to avoid spending months in casts or in surgery after falls that break bones you really need to stay mobile.

You can prevent osteoporosis or at least reduce its severity, but it takes lifestyle changes that start in childhood. Is making the lifestyle changes worth it? Ask anyone who's spent six months recovering from a broken hip. Does it take discipline? Yes — but so does learning to walk again.

Nothing in life is simple, but our goal is to educate you as painlessly as possible to the high cost of osteoporosis, and the newest ways to prevent, diagnose, and treat it. Don't fall into the trap of believing that osteoporosis is inevitable; we're here to help you avoid the bad breaks.

About This Book

We wrote this book hoping it would be less of a "how to" book and more of a "how to avoid" book. In other words, rather than just explain how to deal with osteoporosis, we also want to show how to avoid it altogether.

Unfortunately, for some of you, that's not going to be possible. Some of you already have osteoporosis, and others are inevitably going to have it. For you, we wrote quite a bit of (we hope) helpful information on what medications to take, how to handle a fracture, and how to improve your bone strength.

Osteoporosis is, to a large degree, preventable, but it takes years of planning to prevent it. Although it may be too late to prevent osteoporosis for some of you, others have time — time to educate yourselves, your families, and your friends about building bone that can stand up to the test of time without crumbling.

This book is intended to help you do just that. We wrote it with the personal background of family history of osteoporotic fractures and years of treating patients with osteoporosis. Remember that we didn't write this book to be read all the way through. If you don't have time or if you only want to know about a specific topic, you can go to the section that answers your questions and understand it, without having to read everything that comes before.

However, starting at the beginning may be best for you if you want to know exactly what osteoporosis is. The textbooks say that osteoporosis is "a disease of bony fragility, characterized by low bone mass," but that doesn't really begin to explain the changes your bones undergo when they become osteoporotic. And it certainly doesn't describe the chaos that fragile bones can bring to your life.

Conventions Used in This Book

In this book we use the following conventions to help make everything consistent and easier to understand.

- All Web addresses appear in `monofont`.
- **Bold** text indicates keywords in bulleted lists or highlights the action parts of numbered steps.
- *Italics* identify new terms, followed by an easy-to-understand definition.

What You're Not to Read

Of course we want you to read everything in this book. However, we understand that you may only want to read the essentials. So in this section we identify the "skippable" material if you're in such a hurry that you can't read everything. The following items are interesting to read, but not essential for you to understand and cope with osteoporosis:

- **Text in sidebars:** The sidebars are shaded boxes that appear throughout the book. They sometimes share fun facts, but nothing that's vital to you understanding osteoporosis.
- **Anything with a Technical Stuff icon attached**: This information is interesting, but you won't break a bone if you skip it.
- **The stuff on the copyright page:** Although the Library of Congress may find this text fascinating, we doubt you'll find anything that enthralling in the legal language. Feel free to pass over it.

Foolish Assumptions

When writing this book, we make a few assumptions about you, our dear reader. Those assumptions include the following:

- You or someone you know has been diagnosed with osteoporosis, or you're concerned about osteoporosis prevention.
- You want to know about both osteoporosis prevention *and* treatments.
- You want to know what to expect when you break a bone.
- You want to know how to find the right specialists for treating osteoporosis.
- You want to know how to treat the pain that inevitably accompanies a fracture.

We also assume that when you read each chapter or section, you want quick answers on any number of issues related to osteoporosis. The one theme we thread throughout every chapter and section is that an ounce of prevention is worth a ton of cure.

Osteoporosis isn't inevitable. Fight it hard, with all the tools at your disposal. We hope that one day this book will be obsolete, because osteoporosis will be a disease of the past. And when that day comes, we'll be dancing for joy — or doing some other weight-bearing exercise to strengthen our bones!

How This Book Is Organized

We divide *Osteoporosis For Dummies* into four parts. You don't have to read them in any order. Like any *For Dummies* book, you can skip to what you really need to know at the moment. The following sections explain how we organized this book.

Part I: Understanding Your Bones

This part starts with an explanation of what osteoporosis is, and why it's a serious health problem. We give you a crash course in Bone 101, and describe who gets osteoporosis and why. We review the most common risk factors for osteoporosis and some of the uncommon ones, too. In addition, we talk about the osteoporosis you don't hear much about: osteoporosis in men and kids.

Part II: Keeping Bones Healthy

In these chapters, we give you the best ammunition possible to fight osteoporosis. We also tell you what to eat and what types of exercise build the strongest bones.

Part III: Diagnosing and Treating Osteoporosis

If you have osteoporosis, you want to get to the nitty-gritty: how best to treat it, what the latest and best medications are, what to do if you break a bone, and what the future holds in the diagnosis and treatment of osteoporosis. You can find it all and more in this part.

Part IV: The Part of Tens

Sometimes you need your information in little bites that are lighter and easier to digest. In the Part of Tens chapters, we tell you some great ways to get your daily calcium and enjoy it at the same time, give you ten things you need to know about bones, fill you in on ten great resources for more bone information, and give you some great parenting tips to help encourage your kids to take better care of their bones.

We also share Dr. O'Connor's list of the "questions patients ask most often" about osteoporosis, and give you her answers. It's like a private doctor's visit — without the co-pay!

Icons Used in This Book

Icons are strange little pictures that show up occasionally in the margins in each chapter. We include them to let you know that a topic or a bit of information is special in some way. *Osteoporosis For Dummies* includes the following four icons:

The Tip icon lets you know that you're about to read something helpful that can save you some time or trouble.

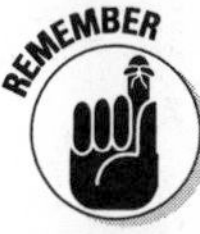

The Remember icon highlights key points of whatever discussion you're reading and points out information that you really need to consider.

Pay close attention to the information that this icon flags. It lets you know that potentially serious trouble or problems may be lurking, but you can avoid the trouble by paying heed to our advice.

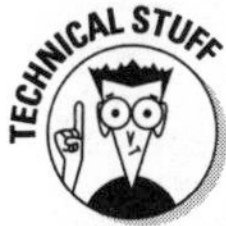

The subject of osteoporosis, of course, often runs into a great deal of medical jargon or study findings. Although you don't need to know this information to tackle the basic issues of osteoporosis, this icon points it out in case you're interested.

Where to Go from Here

We wrote this book to be used as a resource, which means you can pick it up, get a quick answer on whatever's troubling you that day, and put it down without feeling guilty about not reading an entire section. If you're looking for specific information, jumping around is okay.

For example, if you just came home from your doctor's office with a bewildering array of prescriptions, feel free to go straight to Chapter 10. There we describe everything you want to know about prescription medicine commonly prescribed to treat osteoporosis, plus a few things you may not really need to know but that are interesting tidbits.

Are you feeling guilty about your lack of exercise routine and wanting to set up a simple routine that really works without setting a single out-of-shape foot in the gym? Check out Chapter 6. We even give you pictures because it's a lot easier to do an exercise after you see a picture of it.

On the other hand, if you want to discover everything you can about osteoporosis, start reading Chapter 1 and don't stop until you close the book after the appendix. Don't forget to stop for meals and bathroom breaks. Or take a more leisurely approach, and enjoy reading whichever chapter interests you most first. Just like all other *For Dummies* books, you can pick up this book and put it down at will. You can read a chapter a day, a chapter an hour, or a chapter a year and still get the answers you need, when you need them.

Part I

Understanding Your Bones

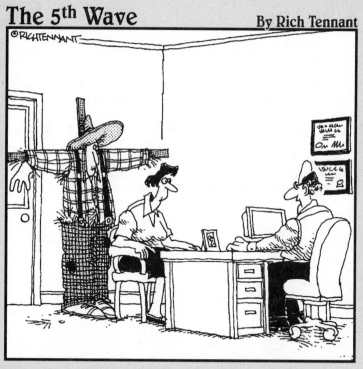

"Your osteoporosis is highly treatable, however, your husband's wood rot will require a whole new stake being shoved down his back."

In this part . . .

Pssst . . . do you want to know all about your bones? Okay, so maybe understanding your bones doesn't sound all that alluring or mysterious. But after you dig up a few bony tidbits, we think you'll agree that bones are complicated and fascinating. In this part, we help you discover where bones come from, what makes them strong, and how you can make yours last a lifetime.

Chapter 1

Boning Up on Osteoporosis

In This Chapter

- Figuring out what osteoporosis really is
- Getting an early diagnosis
- Doing your best to avoid osteoporosis
- Building up your (and your children and grandchildren's) bone density
- Dealing with osteoporosis
- Understanding the difference between osteoporosis and other diseases

Years ago, when your authors first started taking care of patients, doctors had no way to diagnosis early osteoporosis. By the time osteoporosis was apparent on a regular X-ray or a fracture had occurred, significant bone loss had already affected the individual. Nor did doctors have any effective drugs to treat or prevent osteoporosis. We've come a long way, baby, in the early detection, prevention, and treatment of osteoporosis.

In this chapter, we introduce you to the problems of osteoporosis and explain why it's an issue affecting everyone. Even if you're not at risk for developing osteoporosis, you undoubtedly have a younger loved one who is in the process of building bone. We want to help you understand what you can do to make your bones, and those of your loved ones, the best they can be, even if you've never had a glass of milk in your adult life.

Defining Osteoporosis

What exactly is osteoporosis? The standard World Health organization (WHO) definition is that *osteoporosis* is "a skeletal disorder characterized by compromised bone strength predisposing a person to an increased risk of fracture," which is certainly a mouthful, if not a particularly enlightening one. Osteoporosis is the most common bone disease by far, but it's a disease many people don't understand.

Most people think of osteoporosis only in terms of bone fractures or loss of height, but osteoporosis is far more complicated. You'd probably understand osteoporosis most clearly if you could see a bone specimen affected by osteoporosis under the microscope, but you're not likely to ever be privy to a bone biopsy. Doctors don't usually perform bone biopsies in their patients to diagnosis osteoporosis, although pathological examination of bone is still the gold standard in diagnosing osteoporosis. Normal bone has a network of strong plates and bands. In osteoporosis the bands become thinner and weakened, and worse yet there are tiny breaks in the plates and bands.

Another way to define osteoporosis is that osteoporosis is present if bone mineral testing value is more than 2.5 standard deviations below the average adult, even if there's no history of fractures. (See Chapter 9 for more on bone mineral density tests.)

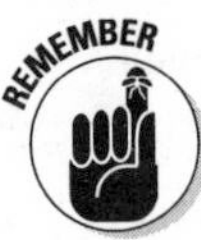

The word "osteoporosis" actually means *porous bones.* If something is porous, it has holes in it. Although all bone has cavities filled with cells and blood (see Chapter 2 for more information on bone biology), in osteoporosis, the normal bony cavities enlarge. When the "holes" become larger, bone becomes more fragile and more susceptible to breaking. Minimal trauma can cause a fracture when you have osteoporosis. Osteoporosis is a systemic disorder that affects the entire skeleton.

Bone is in a constant state of *remodeling;* old bone is broken down and replaced with new bone (see Chapter 2 for more on how bone is built). Osteoporosis can occur when you lose more bone than you rebuild, or when more bone than normal is broken down. (See Chapter 3 for risk factors that are responsible for changes in your bone density.)

Bone mass decreases between 1 and 5 percent per year after age 40 in women, and less than 1 percent in men. Women are more likely to develop osteoporosis because they generally have less bone mass to start with than men do. The sudden loss of *estrogen,* a sex hormone that is instrumental in building healthy bone, in menopause also contributes to women's increased risk of osteoporosis.

Who, Me? How Osteoporosis May Affect You

If you're reading this book, you may already be proactive about your bone health. Maybe you already know that you need to change your diet, exercise more, and take that extra calcium supplement. This book can help those of you who want to prevent osteoporosis. If you already have osteoporosis, this book can explain the ways to treat it and to prevent it from worsening.

To emphasize just how common the problem of osteoporosis is, a recent report from the Surgeon General's office stated that by the year 2020, half of all Americans older than age 50 will be at risk for fractures from osteoporosis. Of women now age 50 or older, 40 percent will suffer a fracture of the hip, wrist, or spine at some point in their lives.

Your co-author Sharon works with a population of patients who are older than 60 years of age. Part of her job includes weighing and measuring each patient. Invariably, nearly every person laments that they used to be taller than they are now. (Thinner too, but that's another issue!)

Losing height used to be considered an inevitable part of aging, similar to wrinkles and age spots. Most people don't realize that one cause of height loss is related to fractures in the spinal column called *vertebral compression fractures.* Between 60 and 70 percent of women older than age 65 have at least one of these fractures.

Even worse, studies show that 20 percent of people with a vertebral fracture will sustain another fracture within a year. And people with compression fractures have a relative risk of death that is nine times higher than their healthy counterparts.

If you're one of the 28 million Americans who currently have osteoporosis, or one of the 18 million who have low bone mass and are likely to develop osteoporosis in the future, don't despair! Even if you've already broken a bone or two, you can take some steps to decrease your odds of fracture in the future. This book can help you implement those changes in your life.

Looking more closely at the numbers: How serious is osteoporosis?

Statistics related to osteoporosis are staggering. Consider just a few from the 2004 Surgeon General's report:

- Around 1.5 million people have a fracture related to osteoporosis each year.
- Hip fractures are responsible for 300,000 hospitalizations each year.

- Up to 700,000 vertebral compression fractures and 250,000 wrist fractures occur in the United States each year.
- The cost for treating osteoporotic fractures each year is around $18 *billion* — $38 million a day.
- Approximately 20 percent of seniors who suffer a hip fracture will die within one year.
- Around 20 percent of seniors with a hip fracture will be in a nursing home within a year.
- White women older than age 65 are twice as likely to fracture something as African American women. Latino women's fracture rates fall between the two groups.

  A woman's risk of hip fracture is equal to her risk of developing breast, uterine, and ovarian cancer combined.
- By the year 2050, men will have one half of all hip fractures in the United States.

Defeating fragility fractures before they occur

You can't see or feel changes in your bone strength over time. In other words, osteoporosis is a disease without warning signs. After you've experienced your first *fragility fracture,* a fracture that occurs after an event that normally wouldn't be traumatic enough to cause a fracture, you've already lost a significant amount of bone density.

Fragility fractures are strong predictors for another fracture in the future. If you have a fragility fracture, you need thorough evaluation and treatment by someone who specializes in osteoporosis (see Chapter 8 for more on choosing a doctor to treat osteoporosis).

The first outward sign of osteoporosis could be a devastating hip fracture or spinal compression fracture. But you can avoid these breaks. How, you may ask?

Your doctor can detect osteoporosis before that first break! A simple new kind of X-ray known as *Dual Energy X-ray Absorptiometry (DXA),* also known as *bone densitometry,* can measure your bone density. Your doctor then uses this information to predict the likelihood of a future fragility fracture. (See Chapter 9 for more information about DXA scans.)

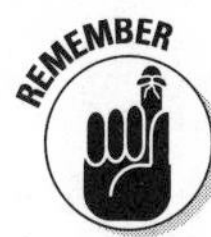

After you've had a baseline bone mineral density test, your doctor may ask you to repeat the test every two years to see how your bones are holding up to the stress of aging.

Uncovering the relationship between aging and osteoporosis

Bones, like Rome, weren't built in a day. It takes years to build up your bone density, and your behaviors, both good and bad, during the time of peak bone development can impact the amount of bone you end up with.

Your bones actually remodel and reshape themselves throughout your lifetime, something that most people don't even notice until something goes wrong. You may wonder why a process that seems to progress painlessly (with any luck at all) from birth to around age 45 suddenly seems to fall apart at the bones, as it were.

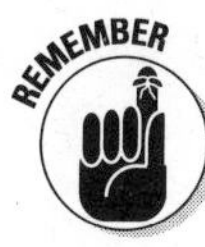

By the time you reach the age of 35 or so, you've amassed all the bone you'll ever have. Several factors, such as heredity, your diet, your exercise levels, and whether you smoke, drink alcohol, or have any other "bad" habits, determine your peak bone mass. (See Chapter 3 for more on determining your risk factors.)

After age 35, you can maintain the bone mass you already have, but you can't increase your peak bone mass. For women, the start of menopause, with its sudden drop in estrogen is the start of accelerated bone loss. For men, bone loss happens later in life. (Check out Chapter 4 for more on men and osteoporosis.)

Suddenly the bone you're building isn't keeping pace with the bone that's being broken down. The various medications used to treat osteoporosis affect this delicate balance. (See Chapter 10 for more on osteoporosis and medications). You can also achieve improvement in bone strength by doing weight-bearing exercises (see Chapter 6) and by taking in enough calcium and vitamin D (see Chapter 5).

Why Early Diagnosis Is So Important

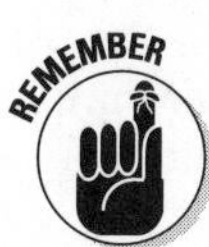

The earlier you start preventing and treating osteoporosis, the better your chances of preserving bone. Waiting until you've broken a bone and then trying to "catch up" on bone strength isn't nearly as effective as building good bone in your early years.

Unfortunately, the peak bone-building years coincide with the years where people sometimes ignore health issues. Given that most 25-year-olds aren't terribly concerned with their bones, the next best way to get people to pay attention to their bones is to diagnose problems early enough to catch and treat little problems before they become big ones.

Keep a close eye on your young children and grandchildren. Even though kids do break bones, it doesn't mean they have osteoporosis. In fact, not all fractures are a fragility fracture. However, a child who breaks several bones within a year needs to be tested for possible bone disease (see Chapter 4 for more on children and osteoporosis), unless the child in question has a propensity for jumping off roofs or otherwise taking increased risks.

If you have known risk factors, such as long-term use of corticosteroids or a strong family history of osteoporosis, don't wait until you're wearing your first cast to find out if you have osteoporosis. Talk to your doctor and ask to have a baseline bone density test, and make sure that your diet includes the recommended amount of calcium and vitamin D for your age group. And don't forget to exercise! (Remember that bone loss occurs every year after menopause unless you're taking steps to prevent it.)

Many situations increase your risk for developing osteoporosis. Knowing some of them can get you started off in the right direction for an early diagnosis and prevention. Some important risk factors are in the following list:

- Chronic illnesses, such as liver or kidney disease
- Chronic use of corticosteroids, such as prednisone
- Difficulty absorbing nutrients due to problems with your stomach or intestines
- Estrogen or testosterone deficiencies
- Excessive use of tobacco or alcohol
- Low body weight
- Periods of immobilization

Improving Your Peak Bone Density — And Your Children's

If more Americans truly practiced prevention instead of searching for a cure after the inevitable has happened, everyone would be a lot healthier.

This statement is as true with osteoporosis as with other diseases. For example, if people spent 1⁄100 of the time trying to build a good peak bone density up to age 25 or 30, many of them wouldn't have to worry about what drug to take to cure their osteoporosis.

Your bone density potential is partly determined by hereditary factors, and partly by environmental factors. Many experts today are especially concerned that today's children are going to suffer from osteoporosis due to a number of problems. What are they?

- Children spend more time sitting (as in front of the computer) and less time exercising.
- Children spend more time indoors and therefore receive less exposure to vitamin D, a vitamin necessary for bones.
- Teenage girls usually have to deal with peer pressure to stay as thin as possible.
- Children are substituting soft drinks for milk.
- More teens are smoking.
- Some teenage girls also exercise too strenuously, attempting to keep weight down or to attain success in weight-driven sports, such as ballet or gymnastics. (See Chapter 4 for more on this condition known as *female athlete triad.*)

Studies show that adolescents who take in less than 1,000 milligrams of calcium daily (boys) and 850 milligrams (girls) of calcium won't achieve their optimal bone mass.

If you're already older than 30, you can try and build strong bones in your children and grandchildren by encouraging them to get up off their bottoms and go outside and run around. (See Chapter 4 for more about children and osteoporosis.) You can feed them — and yourself — nutritious meals and set a good example by drinking your milk. In fact, teens make nearly one-third of their spinal peak bone mass during adolescence, yet their eating habits often aren't focused upon bone building, especially among teenage girls concerned about their weight.

Certainly knowing your family history is important. Look at your family photographs for changes in your relatives' spines. If you know that your grandma and mom both had osteoporosis, make sure that you avoid the dangerous habits of cigarette smoking and excess alcohol consumption.

Evaluating Osteoporosis Therapy

The goal of therapy for osteoporosis is to reduce fractures, because fractures do much more than break bone. Fractures can change a person's life, or possibly end it prematurely. In fact, people who suffer from hip fractures have a higher chance of dying because the surgery increases your risk of getting pneumonia or blood clots in your lungs. The pain and suffering from osteoporosis costs billions of dollars of treatment in the United States alone.

All treatment, whether it be preventive or therapeutic and whether it involves taking medication or just getting up off the couch and exercising, is aimed at preventing fractures caused by weak bones. Unfortunately studies in the United States have shown that many patients who have had a hip fracture weren't tested or treated for osteoporosis.

This book tells you about how doctors can diagnose osteoporosis early and how they can treat osteoporosis. Hence, we're delighted that you've decided to read our book and bone up on osteoporosis, because our goal is to prevent the breaks that can shatter far more than just bone. (Check out Chapter 9 that focuses on testing your bones and Chapter 10 that focuses on different prescription medications to help your osteoporotic bones.)

Terminology 101: Keeping Your "Osteos" Straight

The word "osteo" is derived from the Greek word for *bone.* Many medical conditions and terms start with this same Greek word, and they focus on bones. However, the different "osteo" conditions really have little to do with one another. In this section we try to help you determine the differences between osteoporosis and the other "osteos" you may encounter.

Osteoarthritis: It hurts, but it's not osteoporosis

*Osteo*porosis and *osteo*arthritis are both common conditions in people older than 65, but these two conditions are completely different problems.

Osteoarthritis is a problem that affects your joints. It results from the loss of the cartilage that acts as a cushion between the joints of your bones. Osteoarthritis causes pain in your joints and has nothing to do with osteoporosis, even though both words start with "osteo." Perhaps, if the medical community used the phrase "degenerative joint disease," for osteoarthritis, people wouldn't confuse the two.

More than 20 million Americans have osteoarthritis; before age 45, more men than women have osteoarthritis, but after age 55, osteoarthritis affects more women than men.

The joints most commonly affected in osteoarthritis are certain joints in the fingers, feet, spine, hips, and knees. Repeated trauma to the joints can cause osteoarthritis. Osteoarthritis causes pain and stiffness in the joints; swelling and warmth can also occur. If you have pain and stiffness in your joints after sitting for long periods, you could have osteoarthritis. Sometimes a consultation with a rheumatologist is necessary for confirmation. (Refer to `www.rheumatology.org` to see exactly what a rheumatologist does.)

Treatment for osteoarthritis includes anti-inflammatory drugs, such as ibuprofen (Motrin) and naproxen (Aleve), aspirin, or acetaminophen (Tylenol). Physical therapy, mild exercise, and weight loss, if you're overweight, can also help osteoarthritis.

Osteomalacia: So why exactly did that bone break?

*Osteo*malacia is an illness that also causes fragility fractures, but it's much less common than osteoporosis. If you have a broken bone, you may think quibbling about whether your fracture was caused by osteoporosis or *osteomalacia* is silly. But the treatment for each can be different, so you and your doctor need to know which condition is affecting your bones.

Osteomalacia is primarily a disorder of decreased bone mineralization. Your doctor can diagnose osteomalacia with a bone biopsy or by history, physical examination, laboratory, and radiological studies.

So what exactly are the differences between the two? Osteoporosis usually occurs in a population with certain risk factors; they're postmenopausal women, people older than age 65, or patients who have been on long-term corticosteroid therapy. Osteoporosis patients generally have normal blood levels of calcium, phosphate, vitamin D, and parathyroid hormones, to name a few. Patients with osteomalacia may have low levels of vitamin D, calcium, and phosphates, and high levels of parathyroid hormones.

In osteoporosis, the amount of bone mass you have is reduced, making your bones more porous, but the mineral makeup of the bone is normal. Because the bones have less mass, they're fragile. In osteomalacia, the bones themselves are soft and brittle, because their mineral content is abnormal.

Sometimes the only way to distinguish between osteoporosis and osteomalacia is through a bone biopsy. You can have a bone biopsy as an outpatient procedure; typically your doctor samples a bit of bone from your *iliac crest* (the bony protrusion near your hip just below your waist).

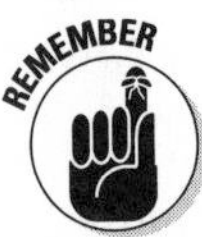

Always remind your doctor to define your problem precisely and consider other causes of reduced bone density.

Osteopenia warning: Falling bone density ahead!

*Osteo*penia is a word that has come to be identified with a numerical reading on your bone density. You have had some bone density loss, but not a lot. It could be a forerunner or warning sign of further bone loss and fractures due to bone loss.

Your doctor can diagnose osteopenia when your bone density tests results show that you have a lower bone density than normal, but not enough to diagnose you with osteoporosis. Dr. O'Connor remembers a time when osteopenia had a different meaning. It meant that your X-rays showed a reduction in bone density. Most doctors don't use osteopenia this way anymore, because they have adapted to the terminology used in reading bone densities.

Understand that osteopenia really doesn't tell you much about why your bone density might be low. It's merely a numerical value obtained from a bone density report.

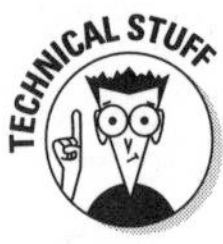

We describe bone density and the ways to test for it more thoroughly in Chapter 9, but a quick way to describe the difference between osteopenia and osteoporosis is that osteopenia is a range of 1 to 2.5 standard deviations below the norm on a bone density test, and anything higher than 2.5 standard deviation is osteoporosis.

Chapter 2

Loving the Living Tissue Called Bone

In This Chapter

- Appreciating that your skeleton is a living organ
- Studying the many functions of bones
- Looking at how the life cycle affects bones
- Exploring how age affects your bones

Bones have a whole life of their own inside you. You may be surprised to discover that your bones are considered an organ similar to a heart or a kidney. In fact, the inside of your bones are constantly changing and being remodeled. Although it may seem that your skeleton is merely an inert support system upon which to hang the rest of your body, this assumption couldn't be farther from the truth.

In this chapter, we discuss the structure, development, and function of bone: the what, why, and how of bone biology otherwise known as BONE 101. Knowing this information can help you understand your bones, how osteoporosis can affect them, and why osteoporosis treatments are designed to do what they do. You need to understand normal bone before you can understand what can go wrong.

Understanding Your Living Skeleton

When most people think of a skeleton, they often think of a Halloween skeleton — inactive with no life. However, similar to all other parts of your body, bone is very much alive, composed of cells and the material made by those cells. In this chapter, we explain why your bone is beautiful. It functions in an amazing way to provide strength and stability for the skeleton; yet, in spite of its strength, it's light and flexible. Bone changes under mechanical stress, it undergoes repair, and it's periodically replaced.

Your co-author Sharon remembers reading a horror story many years ago about a ghoul that sucked the bones out of its victims, leaving them flopping on the ground like helpless, albeit talking, jellyfish. This story is only partly accurate, because without bones people would be very similar to jellyfish, but they would be dead jellyfish, because bones manufacture things that people can't live without.

Bone has so many characteristics. It grows. It remodels itself. It contains a marrow cavity that makes blood cells. Unfortunately, it can break under pressure. At the risk of making you feel as though you're in an anatomy and physiology class, we want you to have a basic understanding of how your bones work. After you understand what makes bones work, you can better understand — and avoid — the problems that prevent bones from doing their job.

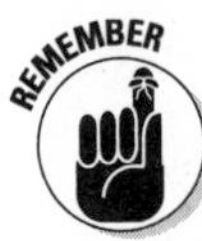

Although bones in your skeleton *look* inert; in reality, they're very busy — all the time. They have a number of functions to carry out to keep you alive and well. Bones provide

- **Agility:** Bones, in conjunction with their closest attachments, muscles and joints, enable you to get off the couch and do some physical activity. (Oh, you've been stuck on the couch for some time? Sorry, but lifting the remote to change the channel doesn't constitute exercise.)
- **Production of blood cells:** Your bone marrow produces important blood cells including red blood cells, platelets, and some white blood cells.
    - *Red blood cells* carry oxygen around your body.
    - *Platelets* help clot your blood and keep you from bleeding to death from a paper cut.
    - *White blood cells* fight off foreign invaders, such as your neighbor's cold germs.
- **Protection:** Bones shield you from things that could hurt your delicate insides, such as flying objects, walls, and even floors. Without bones, your brain would literally be mush, because it would be severely damaged every time you laid down to sleep. Your heart would literally break every time you picked up a "dangerous" object — like your 20-pound grandchild — and held him or her to your chest.

- **Storage:** Think of your bones as a bank that stores vital minerals, such as calcium and phosphorus. For example, your body needs to maintain a constant level of calcium in the blood so that the rest of your cells can function properly. If you have a disease where calcium blood levels drop, the bone architecture serves as a reservoir for calcium.
- **Support:** Your skeletal system is strong enough to support the upright posture, yet not so heavy as to preclude running and walking.

Meeting Your Bones

There's a lot more to your bones than first meets the eye. Most of you, unless you're a surgeon or have ever had a compound fracture, have never actually seen a live human bone. You may have seen a human skeleton at a museum, but the bone you see there looks dry and boring, not to mention inactive.

The bones you see at a museum are dead. *Your* bones are alive, and if you could get a bird's-eye view of all the cellular-level activity taking place every day, you would have new respect for your bones. They're more productive than any factory on the planet!

You're not freaky: Looking at unusual bones

Most of you have the same number of bones, which is 206. (Did you remember that number or did you have to pull out your high school biology notes?) But some of you may be lucky enough to have a few extra here and there. Extra bones are generally one of two types: *Wormian* (also known as *sutural,* which certainly sounds nicer) and *sesmoid* bones.

- **Wormian bones** are small clusters of bones found between the joints of some cranial bones.
- **Sesmoid bones** are in tendons in areas of pressure, such as the wrist or ankle. Not to confuse you too much, but one type of sesmoid bone, the *patella,* or kneecap, is normally found in everybody.

Your co-author Sharon knows sesmoid bones well. She had one removed from her foot after it caused recurring tendonitis and made walking from point A to point B difficult. The tendency to have extra bones is hereditary, and almost everyone in Sharon's family has this same extra bone in the same place.

Looking at the different types of bones

Although bones contain the same basic structure, they differ in appearance and function. Generally, two types of tissue comprise bones:

- **Cortical:** Also called compact bone, cortical bone is dense.
- **Trabecular:** Also called spongy bone, trabecular bone is lightweight and porous, because it contains many little holes.

Most bones contain both cortical and trabecular tissue. Check out "Examining the innards and outards of your bones" later in this chapter for more on cortical and trabecular bones.

Furthermore, bones fall into four different category types, listed and defined in the following bulleted list.

- **Long bones** are merely longer than they are wide, but they aren't necessarily all that long. Some of the bones in fingers and toes are long bones even though they're really fairly short. Other long bones, such as the femur in your thigh and the humerus in your arm, are fairly long. Long bones are composed of mostly cortical bone.
- **Short bones** are actually more cube shaped. Most short bones consist of trabecular tissue. Your wrist and ankle contain short bones.
- **Flat bones** are thin and provide protection to underlying important parts like your brain and heart. Ribs, sternum, and shoulder blades are all flat bones. So is your skull. Trust us on this one. Although your skull is curved, it's made out of flat bones. Flat bones are generally cortical bone with a spongy center.
- **Irregular bones** are bones that don't fit in any other category, like your vertebrae and some of your facial bones. Irregular bones are mostly made up of trabecular tissue.

Examining the innards and outards of your bones

Cortical bone surrounds bones and makes up 75 percent of your total skeletal mass. The bone inside the shell, trabecular bone, is composed of plates and rods that are arranged in a network of patterns that provide maximum strength with minimum bulk. (See Figure 2-1.) Most bones contain both types of tissue, but the proportions may vary from bone to bone. Cortical bone predominates in your arms, ribs, and legs. It also regenerates itself rather slowly, about 2 to 3 percent a year.

You primarily find trabecular bone in the spine, pelvis, and hip. The relative hollowness of trabecular bone makes it more vulnerable to certain problems related to bone metabolism, such as osteoporosis, hyperparathyroidism, or calcium deficiencies. (See Chapter 7 for further discussion of metabolic bone diseases.) Trabecular bone makes up about 20 percent of your bone mass and regenerates more rapidly than cortical bone — about 25 percent a year compared to 3 percent for cortical bone.

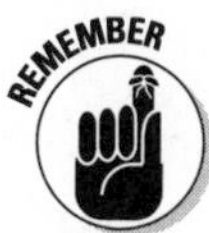

Over the course of a lifetime, women may lose about 40 percent and men between 15 and 40 percent of their trabecular bone. Women lose 30 to 40 percent of cortical bone, while men lose 5 to 15 percent.

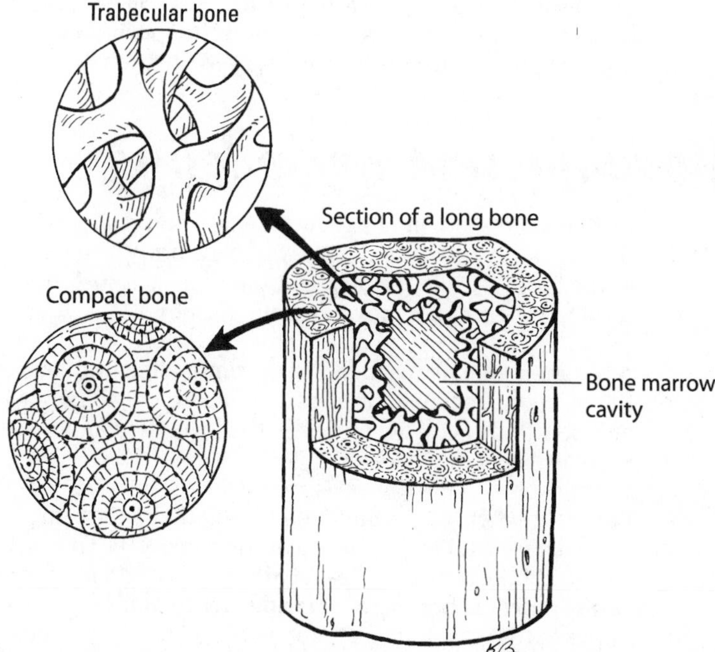

Figure 2-1: Bones contain two types of bone tissue: trabecular and cortical, or compact. Compact bone is the dense outer shell, whereas trabecular bone is the lighter inner portion of bone.

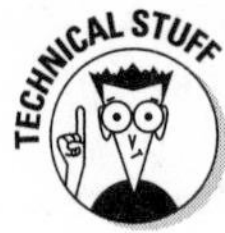

Chemically speaking, all bone is composed of a crystal-like structure that is bound to proteins. These crystals are composed of minerals (predominately calcium and phosphorus) arranged in an orderly structure referred to as *hydroxyapatite*. These crystals are bound to the protein matrix that is composed primarily of collagen molecules.

Although you may think of collagen as primarily a magic substance to plump up lips or send wrinkles to never-neverland, collagen is actually a protein that works as the "foundation" that holds your skin, tendon, bone, cartilage, and connective tissue together. There are several types of collagen. The major collagen in bone is type I collagen.

This composition provides both strength and resiliency. Another way of thinking about this is to imagine a scaffold (consisting of cross-linked collagen molecules) upon which crystals are deposited in an orderly fashion.

There can be problems with collagen formation. For example, when the body makes abnormal type I collagen molecules, a severe genetic form of osteoporosis, known as *osteogenesis imperfecta,* can result. See Chapter 7 for more information on this illness. When there are problems in the way minerals deposit on bone, another bone problem called *osteomalacia* (see Chapter 1) can develop.

Modeling and Remodeling

During childhood, bones grow in length and change their shapes through a process called *modeling*. New bone forms on the outside of the cortex, while the inside of the bone is *resorbed* (a special term that refers to removal of bone tissue).

After a person has reached her maximum height, the process continues so that small injuries can be repaired. Old bone is removed and new bone is made; however, the formation and resorption are more closely coupled.

Basically, when you're an adult, during the remodeling process, bone is removed and replaced at the same site. This occurs on the surface of the *trabecule* (trabecular bone) or on the inside of the *cortex* (cortical bone). An amazing fact to mull over about your bones is that the adult skeleton is completely replaced every ten years!

Now that you have some knowledge of how your bones are structured, to further understand how this information deals with osteoporosis, you need to know three important pieces: what builds up bones, what breaks them down, and what keeps the breaking down and building up in balance. The next section explains these processes.

Building Up and Breaking Down: Your Bones Day by Day

As we state earlier in the chapter, bone is constantly reshaping itself in a complex process of building and remodeling. You don't notice this reshaping because it happens on a microscopic level. The major players involved in bone building and remodeling are

- **The cells:** Osteoblasts, osteoclasts, and osteocytes
- **The hormones:** The directors of cellular function
- **The essential minerals**: Most commonly calcium and phosphorus

Blasts, clasts, and cytes (oh my)

An intricate balance between the activities of two major cell types referred to as the osteoblast and osteoclast determine a person's total bone mass.

An easy way to remember the work of osteoblasts, osteoclasts, and osteocytes is

> Osteoblasts giveth.
>
> Osteoclasts taketh away.
>
> Osteocytes maintaineth.

Osteoblasts are the builders and make collagen and hydroxyapatite. Some of the osteoblasts become buried in their matrix and then they are referred to as *osteocytes.* The rest of the osteoblasts cover the new bone's surface (see Figure 2-2). Waves of osteoblasts that move into the area form new layers of bone.

Osteoclasts are larger cells whose function is to dissolve bone by acting on the mineral matrix. They make enzymes such as *collagenase,* which breaks down collagen. Osteoclasts also secrete various acids that can dissolve the hydroxyapatite structure.

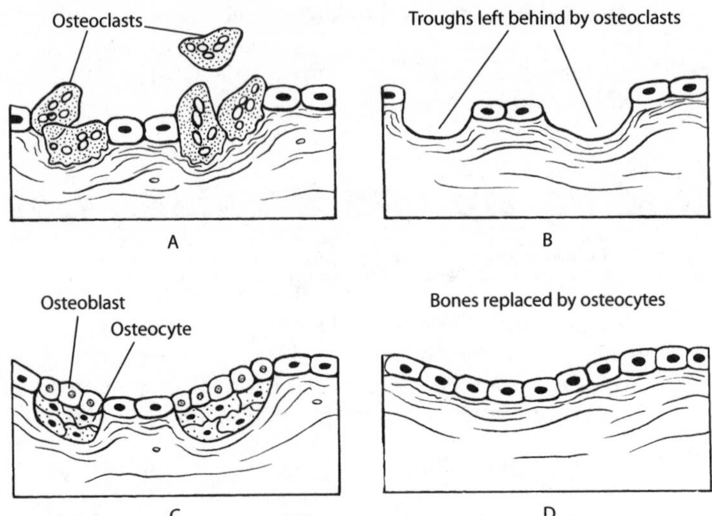

Figure 2-2: Osteoblasts build up bone; osteoclasts break down bone.

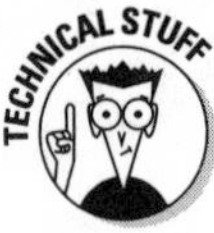

There are a variety of signals that control the function of osteoblasts and osteoclasts. Interestingly, osteoblasts make small proteins, one of which is called OPG (osteoprotegrin). OPG can prevent osteoclasts from being activated. Osteoblasts change their shape and become buried in their matrix, connected to each other only by thin processes called *canaliculi.* After the osteoblasts are buried in bone, they're referred to as osteocytes. Osteocytes account for 90 percent of all cells in the skeleton.

Bone remodeling starts with resorption, which the osteoclasts orchestrate. Osteoclasts break down bone by dissolving mineral and resorbing the matrix that osteoblasts have formed. Refer to Figure 2-2.

More research into the function of these cells will undoubtedly result in new drugs to treat osteoporosis. Scientists now understand that the process of building up bone and resorption of bone is critical because abnormalities in these processes lead to bone diseases.

Fine-tuning your bones with hormones

Hormones are the directors of the entire process of keeping bone in proper balance. Many hormones contribute to the balance, but the hormones in this section are the most important.

Vitamin D

Vitamin D is a critical hormone that you need for proper bone mineralization. The body mainly absorbs it through your skin from sunlight, although you do absorb some through the stomach by way of diet and supplements.

When vitamin D is absorbed in the skin, it's an inactive hormone and requires special changes that occur in both the kidney and liver. Certain drugs interfere with vitamin D metabolism and therefore cause soft fragile bone. Vitamin D deficiency can also occur from a poor diet and lack of exposure to sunlight.

Vitamin D has many important functions in addition to its role in mineralization. For example, vitamin D helps to maintain normal blood levels of calcium by promoting calcium absorption in the intestine. Hence, vitamin D helps keep bones from becoming thin, brittle, or misshapen. An adequate amount of vitamin D (see Chapter 5 for more on vitamin D in foods) in your diet or through vitamin D supplements prevents rickets in children (see Chapter 4 for more on rickets) and *osteomalacia,* a condition where bones are soft and brittle, in adults. (Refer to Chapter 11 on taking vitamin D supplements.)

Parathyroid hormone (PTH)

Parathyroid hormone (also known as PTH) is another key director. The parathyroid gland, which is actually a set of four small glands located near your thyroid gland, produces this hormone.

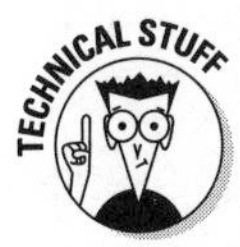

PTH provides for the exquisite regulation of calcium metabolism. For example, when the serum level of calcium drops, the parathyroid gland synthesizes more hormone. PTH instructs the kidney to hold onto more calcium. It also directs how much calcium is allowed to be stored in the bone.

Basically, PTH is the traffic director of calcium, regulating how much calcium you absorb with your diet, how much calcium your kidneys secrete, and how much calcium your bones store. Osteoblasts have receptors for PTH. When these receptors are activated, the osteoblasts make less OPG. This small molecule in turn regulates the activity of osteoclasts.

Calcitonin

Calcitonin, a hormone produced by the thyroid gland, inhibits bone removal by osteoclasts, and promotes bone formation by osteoblasts. Calcitonin is also one of the older drugs used to treat osteoporosis. (See Chapter 10 for more on drugs that treat osteoporosis.)

Estrogen

Estrogen is a hormone that is instrumental in regulating women's menstrual cycles. Estrogen also works with the parathyroid glands to keep calcium levels in balance. The drop in estrogen levels at menopause is one of the reasons why women begin to develop osteoporosis.

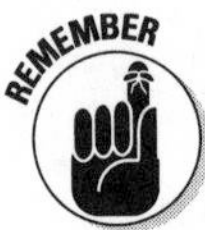

Estrogen deficiency is one of the most important factors in the development of bone fragility. For some reason, estrogen deficiency results in the production of more osteoclasts and more active osteoclasts. (Check out Chapter 10 for more on estrogen.)

Testosterone

Although you may associate the hormone testosterone with men, both men and women produce testosterone. Testosterone helps maintain strong bone and muscles, and stimulates bone formation. Testosterone deficiency clearly is associated with osteoporosis. (Refer to Chapter 10 for more on testosterone.)

Orchestrating bone growth with minerals

The two most important minerals your body needs to orchestrate bone growth are calcium and phosphorus. Calcium is the most common mineral found in your body and contributes to bone strength. Remember that the crystal hydroxyapatite is composed of calcium. (Check out "Examining the innards and outards of your bones" earlier in this chapter for more about hydroxyapatite.)

Osteoblasts add calcium to your bones, and doctors don't completely understand just how the crystals are formed. Osteoclasts remove calcium from your bones. In fact, an interesting tidbit: The 206 bones in your body contain about three pounds of calcium! Also, remember that when the rest of your body needs calcium, the bone tissue will supply it and the integrity of your bones may suffer as a result!

Phosphorus is the second most important mineral found in your body, because it's the other major component of hydroxyapatite.

Your bones and teeth store approximately 85 percent of the phosphorus.

Phosphorus and calcium work together to build healthy bones. Your body attempts to achieve a balanced ratio of calcium to phosphorus. When this balance is disrupted, various bone diseases can result. Too little or too much phosphorus is harmful. Many other cells use phosphorus, like calcium, to keep you healthy.

Although an adequate amount of phosphorus is not only good but also essential to getting through the day, an excess amount of phosphorus can be detrimental. A diet high in phosphorus, such as a high-protein diet or a high intake of soft drinks, can decrease calcium in your bones because the excess phosphorus looks for calcium to bind to, removing it from bone if necessary. Many American diets contain too much phosphorus in sodas and not enough calcium.

Your Bones from Birth to Infinity: More Stuff to Know

Did you know that babies actually have more bones than adults do, because some of their bones haven't fused yet and can be counted as two or three? Most adults have 206 bones, but your bones at birth numbered more than 300! Babies and young children also have somewhat bendable bones, so they may have more *greenstick fractures,* which are breaks that occur when bones bend but don't break completely.

This section includes a few more interesting tidbits to know about your bones:

- Bones continue to grow in length and breadth until your late teens or early 20s. Hence bone biologists have developed the term "peak bone mass." This phrase refers to the amount of bony tissue present at the end of skeletal maturation. Your peak bone mass increases throughout adolescence and then peaks in your early 30s. It plateaus for a while and then (for women) starts to decline after menopause. Men start to decline in their 60s. (You can read more about men and osteoporosis in Chapter 4.)

  Factors such as your genetic makeup, nutrition, and activity determine your peak bone mass. Various diseases also can affect your peak bone mass. Understanding the factors that determine peak bone mass are critical in determining ways to prevent osteoporosis, because if you can build stronger bones, even though some bone is lost during aging, you may not have enough bone loss to result in osteoporosis. (Check out Chapter 3 for more discussion on risk factors.)

Your peak bone mass is represented in Figure 2-3 by a bone density measurement. These graphs are different for men and women and are different for different races. This data comes from a large epidemiological study referred to as the National Health and Nutrition Examination Survey (NHANES).

After you've achieved your peak height, your bones continue to remodel on the inside surfaces. In fact, osteoclasts and osteoblasts keep doing their thing. So, if the balance of breaking down and building up is disturbed, you can lose some bone mass.

- Bones respond to forces placed upon them. For example, an athlete who uses his right arm far more often than his left, will develop thicker cortical bone on the right side when compared to the left.

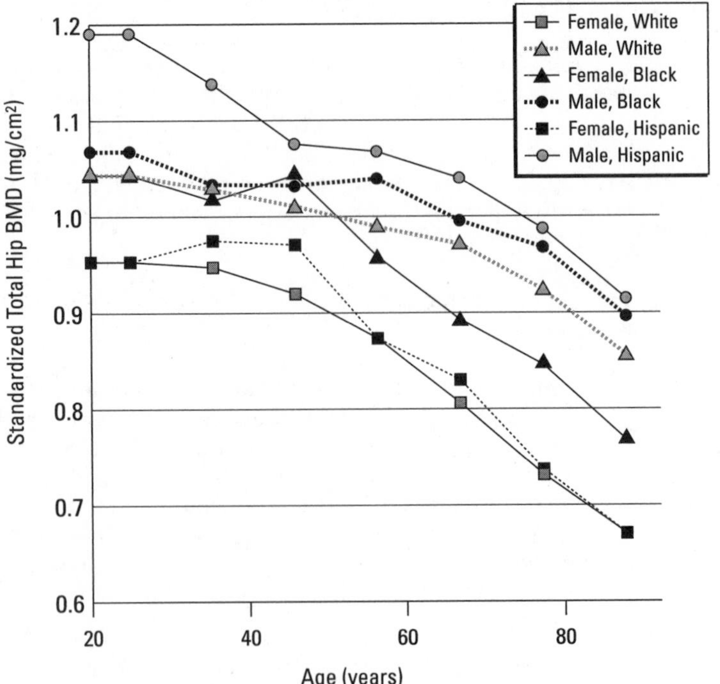

Figure 2-3: Standard bone density measurements determined by age, sex, and race.

- Bone mass is often compared to a bank account. Up until a certain age you're putting more in than you're taking out. But as you age, your withdrawals begin to exceed your deposits, and you begin to lose bone.
- In women, bone loss accelerates after menopause because estrogen levels drop. Women who go through menopause at an earlier age, due to chemotherapy or hormonal disorders, are at higher risk for osteoporosis because they have fewer years to benefit from the protective effects of estrogen.

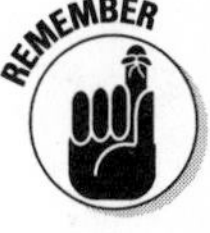

After you reach menopause and lose the protective benefit of higher estrogen levels, your bone withdrawals increase dramatically. You can lose as much as 5 percent of your bone mass each year during the first five years of menopause.

- Men also lose bone mass as they age, but at a much slower rate, normally 0.2 to 0.5 percent per year.

Chapter 3

Breaking Down the Risk Factors

In This Chapter

- Figuring out why women get most of the breaks
- Looking at your lifestyle
- Identifying medications and conditions associated with osteoporosis
- Understanding why certain intestinal problems can increase your risk
- Spotting other diseases related to osteoporosis
- Eyeing ways to lower the risks

Although men do get osteoporosis (see Chapter 4 for more on men and osteoporosis), many more women have osteoporosis. In fact, just being female is your highest risk for osteoporosis. But other factors — family history, your medical history, and your habits, good and bad, also affect your chance of developing osteoporosis, whether you're male or female.

To predict the likelihood of developing osteoporosis, you may be tempted to focus mainly on family history, assuming that if your 90-year-old grandmother is still taller than you are and has better posture than you have, your chances of developing osteoporosis are slim. On the other hand, if your female relatives have owned more walkers, canes, and casts than the average medical supply store, you may believe that you're also destined to experience fractures due to weak bones.

Although family history is important, it's only one factor that determines how likely you are to develop osteoporosis. Both heredity and environment are important when assessing — and reducing — your risk. In this chapter, we compile all the factors that contribute to osteoporosis in women, from hereditary and lifestyle factors to medications and medical conditions.

Assessing Your Risk Factors: Which Women Get Osteoporosis?

Many factors can contribute to your chances of developing osteoporosis. Some factors you can influence, some you can't. In this section, we look at the most common risk factors and what you can do to modify them.

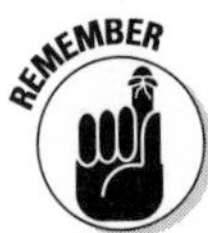

Your doctor can evaluate your chances of having low bone density based on your risk factors and request specialized testing to screen you for osteoporosis *before* you actually get a fracture. (See Chapter 9 for the specifics on testing.)

I am woman, see me shrink

When it comes to osteoporosis, being female is a definite black mark. Men start with more bone mass, and they also lose bone at a slower rate than women. In fact, according to the National Osteoporosis Foundation (NOF), 80 percent of osteoporosis sufferers are women.

Moreover, according to the American Medical Association (AMA), between 20 and 30 percent of women who have gone through menopause have osteoporosis, and another 30 percent have low bone density. If you add up the percentages, you realize that the vast majority of women are at risk. For 8 million women, osteoporosis is a fact, and for another 15 million, it's a looming possibility.

Why do women get all the breaks (so to speak)? In part, the risk is due to normally thinner bones, and partly because the loss of estrogen at menopause accelerates bone loss, especially for the first five to seven years.

So, the biggest single risk factor for developing osteoporosis is simply being female. And, of course, your gender is one thing about yourself that is impossible to change.

Aging is such sweet sorrow

Another unchangeable risk of osteoporosis is age. As difficult as it is to accept, getting older brings not only wrinkles but also the possibility of osteoporosis. Up until her mid-30s, a woman builds more bone than she loses. But after age 35, bone withdrawals start to deplete her bone credit account. Here are several interesting statistics from the AMA about age and bone fractures:

- One out of two women older than 50 will have a bone fracture related to osteoporosis.
- A 50-old woman has a 14 percent risk of hip fracture over the remainder of her lifetime.
- Ninety-plus percent of hip fractures in elderly women are due to osteoporosis.
- One out of five women older than age 50 with a hip fracture will die within one year.

Other factors, however, make some women's risk greater than others. Similar to age and gender, some can't be changed. Others, such as habits, both good and bad, can be. We take a look at both in the next sections.

Blaming it on the family

So the specific question is exactly where do you come from? That's not just a question for your genealogy search; it's an important issue to assess in determining your odds of having osteoporosis.

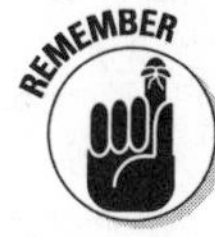

Do you remember when you used to look up to your mom, and now you're looking down on her head instead? Loss of height is a sign of osteoporosis, and a good way to tell if this disease runs in your family — just look through the family album and see if great-grandma got shorter every year. Osteoporosis can be a family affair; if a close female relative had fractures related to osteoporosis, your risks of having osteoporosis are increased, especially if osteoporosis occurred on your mother's side of the family.

It can be frightening to look through a series of pictures and realize that your loved one has become a fraction of her former self; you may start worrying about how many inches you might lose if you develop osteoporosis. Those of you who are short to begin with worry especially about getting shorter! The truth is that a person can lose up to eight inches of height from *vertebral compression fractures,* or fractures of the spine. Average height loss is around three inches. (See Chapters 7 and 13 for more on vertebral compression and other types of fractures.)

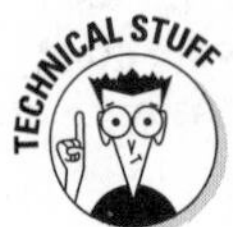

Researchers have been conducting extensive genetic studies to further identify genes that predispose to lower peak bone mineral density and accelerated bone loss in menopause. Perhaps in years to come, DNA testing in adolescence can accurately predict the risk.

But for now, researchers can only rely on some results about who is more predisposed to osteoporosis. Here are some of the more interesting findings:

- Caucasian and Asian women, on average, have bone density 5 to 10 percent lower than women of African American, Mediterranean, or Latino descent. This statistic doesn't mean that only Caucasian and Asian women develop osteoporosis, just that their risk is higher overall.
- Are you a blonde or redhead? (No, we're not going to tell a blonde joke!) Women with fair skin and light hair are also at higher risk for developing osteoporosis. Thin women with narrow hips also have a higher risk of osteoporosis. (We discuss weight in the next section).
- Does premature gray hair run in your family? Some studies have indicated that people who start to go gray in their 20s, and are more than 50 percent gray by age 40, have a higher risk of having osteoporosis.

Don't worry too much. Just because you were blonde in your 20s, turned gray prematurely in your 30s, and are a 100-pound Caucasian doesn't mean you're going to get osteoporosis. You just have a higher risk. As a precaution, talk with your doctor about taking calcium and vitamin D supplements. Discuss with your doctor your risks for osteoporosis. He can advise you on further treatment. (See Chapter 11 for info on supplements.)

Weighty issues

If you're a small and narrow-hipped size two, it's likely that you haven't achieved as high a peak bone density as women who are heavier. Small, thin women generally have small, thin bones, and are more prone to osteoporosis fractures. Some studies are even more specific and say that if you weigh less than 127 pounds at any height, you're prone to osteoporosis.

We remember broken bones: Our personal family histories

One of your co-author Sharon's earliest memories of her maternal great-grandmother was the cast on her arm. She had one of the commonest fractures of osteoporosis, a broken wrist, (in medical lingo: a *Colles'* fracture). Years later, Sharon's children remember *their* great-grandma, daughter of the first, using a walker after she broke her hip. She also lost more than six inches of height due to vertebral compression fractures (fractures of the spine).

Dr. O'Connor's history is a little different. Her father's mother (her paternal grandmother) suffered from painful spinal fractures, followed by a hip fracture. Her son, Dr. O'Connor's dad, had reduced bone density on a scan when he was in his 60s. He was evaluated by a specialist in bone disease and found to have an inherited defect of calcium metabolism called *hypercalciuria,* which can be treated with diuretics (water pills). It's likely that his mother also had hypercalciuria. Always check out your family tree!

Although being naturally small and thin is a risk factor in itself, dieting during adolescence seems to increase your risk of osteoporosis. Excessive dieting may lead to inadequate calcium intake; most research shows that calcium is essential for building normal bone during childhood and adolescence.

Women with a history of anorexia nervosa or bulimia are especially at risk for osteoporosis, according to some studies. They may be two to three times as prone to bone fractures, and the risk may persist throughout their lifetime, if peak bone mass was affected. (See Chapter 4 for more on anorexia and bulimia.)

If you diet or exercise excessively, your menstrual periods may stop altogether. When this happens, you may also develop an estrogen deficiency. In extreme cases, even young women can develop osteoporosis and fractures (see more about osteoporosis in adolescents in Chapter 4).

Your body mass index (BMI) is one way of assessing your risk by weight. (BMI is a formula that takes your height and weight to estimate your body fat.) A body mass index of 20 or less is associated with an increased risk of osteoporosis. See Table 3-1.

Table 3-1 Body Weight in Pounds According to Height and Body Mass Index

BMI(kg/m²)	*19*	*20*	*21*	*22*	*23*	*24*	*25*	*26*	*27*	*28*	*29*	*30*	*35*	*40*
Height (in.)						Weight (lb.)								
58	91	96	100	105	110	115	119	124	129	134	138	143	167	191
59	94	99	104	109	114	119	124	128	133	138	143	148	173	198
60	97	102	107	112	118	123	128	133	138	143	148	153	179	204
61	100	106	111	116	122	127	132	137	143	148	153	158	185	211
62	104	109	115	120	126	131	136	142	147	153	158	164	191	218
63	107	113	118	124	130	135	141	146	152	158	163	169	197	225
64	110	116	122	128	134	140	145	151	157	163	169	174	204	232
65	114	120	126	132	138	144	150	156	162	168	174	180	210	240
66	118	124	130	136	142	148	155	161	167	173	179	186	216	247

BMI(kg/m²)	***19***	***20***	***21***	***22***	***23***	***24***	***25***	***26***	***27***	***28***	***29***	***30***	***35***	***40***
Height (in.)							**Weight (lb.)**							
67	121	127	134	140	146	153	159	166	172	178	185	191	223	255
68	125	131	138	144	151	158	164	171	177	184	190	197	230	262
69	128	135	142	149	155	162	169	176	182	189	196	203	236	270
70	132	139	146	153	160	167	174	181	188	195	202	207	243	278
71	136	143	150	157	165	172	179	186	193	200	208	215	250	286
72	140	147	154	162	169	177	184	191	199	206	213	221	258	294
73	144	151	159	166	174	182	189	197	204	212	219	227	265	302
74	148	155	163	171	179	186	194	202	210	218	225	233	272	311
75	152	160	168	176	184	192	200	208	216	224	232	240	279	319
76	156	164	172	180	189	197	205	213	221	230	238	246	287	328

Women who are overweight have a lower risk of osteoporosis because fat cells produce estrogen. But not many people would consider becoming overweight just to reduce the risk of osteoporosis, especially when being overweight is associated with so many other risk factors. If you're beginning to see controlling your weight to prevent osteoporosis as a no-win situation, you're partially right! However, other risk factors do exist that are more easily adjusted, as you can see in the "Focusing on Lifestyle Factors" later in this chapter.

Starting and stopping menstrual periods

The age when you had your first period and the age when you had your last period are both contributors to your risk of osteoporosis. Estrogen rises during your menstrual cycle, and estrogen helps protect against osteoporosis.

So if your periods started when you were 12, and stopped when you were 50, you got more estrogen over the years than someone whose periods began when she was 16 and stopped when she was 40. You may not have thought at the time that your period was good, but your bones appreciate all that extra estrogen exposure. (See Chapter 10 for more on estrogen replacement therapy in osteoporosis.)

Focusing on Lifestyle Factors

You may not be able to change your height or the (natural!) color of your hair, but you can change some behaviors or habits that can increase your risk of developing osteoporosis. We discuss three of the most important in the next sections.

Smoking and osteoporosis

You know that smoking is bad for your lungs, but did you also know that smoking is bad for your bones? Thinking that smoking, a habit that many people want to quit because of the well-known effects on your lungs, can also be dangerous for your bones may be farfetched, but the facts in the following list make it crystal clear. Studies have shown that

- Smoking decreases the level of estrogen in women. Estrogen helps keep bone healthy.

- Women who smoke go through menopause at an earlier age; estrogen levels drop during menopause.
- Smokers may absorb calcium poorly; calcium is necessary to build strong bones.
- Smoking effects may begin in adolescent smokers; they may have lower than normal bone mass and smaller bone size.
- Fractures heal more slowly in smokers — true of women *and* men.
- By age 80, smokers have bone density 6 to 10 percent lower than nonsmokers.
- Up to one in eight hip fractures in women can be attributed to decrease in bone density due to smoking.
- Estrogen replacement therapy in menopause is less likely to be effective in smokers than nonsmokers.

Although studies may differ on some points, the overall evidence is clear. One of the best preventive measures you can take for your bones is to never start smoking. But if you're already a smoker, try to quit. If you can't quit, at least cut down. Your bones will thank you! (If you need help to stop smoking, check out *Quitting Smoking For Dummies* by David Brizer, MD [Wiley].)

How alcohol affects your bones

When the subject turns to drinking alcohol and osteoporosis, the information is somewhat confusing. Studies show that a moderate intake of alcohol is good for your bones, but that heavy alcohol use is bad for your bones. How do you know what's "too much" and what's "just right" when it comes to alcohol and your bones?

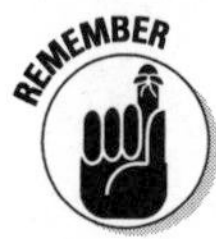

The U.S. Department of Health and Human Services defines "moderate" drinking as one drink per day for women and no more than two drinks a day for men. A single drink is defined as 1.5 ounces of 80 proof distilled spirits, for example, 12 ounces of beer, or 5 ounces of wine. So having a glass of wine — red or white, it's up to you — a day may have benefits for your bones.

One study showed that postmenopausal women who drank 16 drinks a week had a 5 to 10 percent higher bone mass density (BMD) than postmenopausal women who drank less than two drinks per week. This increase in bone density may be because alcohol can help convert testosterone to estrogen after menopause. Alcohol may also increase *calcitonin,* a hormone that inhibits bone resorption, in menopausal women.

What you can't see *can* hurt you

Alcohol can change your body's calcium balance in several ways. Alcohol affects the body in several ways including:

- Alcohol can cause a vitamin D deficiency, which can lead to decreased calcium absorption.
- Alcohol can increase levels of parathyroid hormone (PTH), which puts a strain on your body's calcium reserves.
- Alcohol can increase magnesium excretion, which also decreases bone health.
- Alcohol also suppresses bone formation by its toxic effect on *osteoblasts,* the cells that build bone, and increases bone breakdown by stimulating the formation of *osteoclasts,* the cells that break down bone. (See Chapter 2 for more about bone formation, osteoblasts, and osteoclasts.)

Heavy alcohol consumption also leads to high levels of cortisol, which causes decreased bone formation and impairs calcium absorption by increasing PTH.

However, excessive drinking, especially during adolescence and young adulthood, can decrease bone growth and increase one's risk for developing osteoporosis later in life — true for both men and women. Even more disturbing is the fact that studies have shown that the effects of heavy alcohol at a young age can cause lifelong damage to your overall health, not just to your bones.

If you haven't gone through menopause yet, heavy drinking may cause your periods to be irregular or to stop altogether, decreasing your estrogen levels. Adult women older than 67 years old who drank more than 3 ounces of alcohol a day (the equivalent of six drinks) had greater bone loss than women who drank very little alcohol.

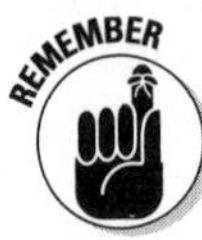

Of course, heavy alcohol intake also puts you at risk for one of the biggest causes of bone fracture: falling!

Watching what you eat

We understand that watching what you eat is no fun. Even though most people would eat a reasonably balanced diet even if they weren't constantly deluged with information on how what they eat affects their health, some people would subsist mostly on cookies and fast food if left to their own devices. This section is for you (and you know who you are!).

Nutrition is so important to bone growth that we devote an entire chapter to it (see Chapter 5). But we also want to throw in a few tidbits here to demonstrate the very real connection between what goes into your mouth and healthy bones.

Women older than 50 need at least 1,500 mg of calcium each day, which is about 4 glasses of fortified milk (6 to 8 ounces per glass) a day. (A glass of milk contains about 400 mg of calcium.) See Chapter 5 for more on calcium intake.

Equally as important to ingesting enough calcium is to make sure you're not losing calcium from poor dietary habits. Some calcium robbers include

- **High animal protein diet:** High protein intake may increase the amount of calcium excreted in your urine. Vegetables and fruit, on the other hand, increase your potassium and magnesium intake, which builds calcium stores. Is the current low-carb diet craze going to be bad news for women down the road? One way to prevent bone loss is to make sure to eat enough veggies in addition to high protein and also to maintain your calcium intake at 1,200 to 1,500 mg a day.
- **Too much salt:** A heavy hand on the saltshaker can result in extra calcium loss.
- **Sodas:** Recent studies indicate that drinking dark colas daily may result in lower bone density. Both regular and diet sodas may have this negative affect on your bones. This loss doesn't occur when phosphoric acid is consumed in foods that also contain calcium. And, of course, if you're drinking soda, you're not drinking something good for you — like milk or calcium-fortified juice. Sodas that contain caffeine may also increase urine output, which can wash away vital mineral stores.

Recognizing Medications That Cause Bone Loss

Many commonly prescribed medications are a double-edged sword for everyone, male or female. On one hand, they cure or help control serious health problems; on the other hand, the medications themselves can cause serious health problems.

Several commonly prescribed medications can increase your chance of developing osteoporosis. Although we're not suggesting that you stop taking medications that can damage your bones, we *are* suggesting that you educate yourself about your medication's side effects. You can take certain precautions, with your doctor and pharmacist's help, to decrease your risk of medication-related osteoporosis.

Why corticosteroids can thin bones

People commonly take *corticosteroids,* such as prednisone, to decrease inflammation in the body, from their eyes to their intestines. If you have serious asthma, an autoimmune disease, severe allergies, or arthritis, you may be taking corticosteroids every day. Corticosteroids help many people live normal lives.

But corticosteroids are very potent medications with the following serious side effects:

- They increase calcium loss through your urine.
- They decrease calcium absorption through your intestinal tract.
- They inhibit growth of new bone.
- They lower estrogen and testosterone hormone levels.

Corticosteroids come in many different forms and under different brand names. No matter how people take corticosteroids, all routes lead to bone loss. (Some people inhale them for asthma and other lung diseases, some inject them, some take them by mouth, and others apply them as creams.)

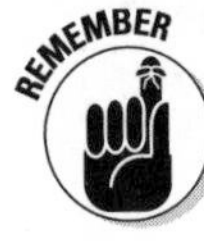

The higher the dose of corticosteroid and the longer the time you take it, the more likely you are to develop osteoporosis. One quarter of all people who take corticosteroids for five to ten years will suffer a fracture. Some studies have shown that you may lose up to 30 percent of bone mass after taking corticosteroids for a relatively short time.

If you absolutely must take corticosteroids of any type long term, doing the following is important:

- Be on the lowest dose possible.
- Reduce your dose slowly. Stopping or reducing your dose too quickly can be dangerous.

- Have your bone density tested every other year, or more frequently if suggested by your doctor.
- For men, check your testosterone levels.
- Check your urine calcium.
- Discuss your concern about osteoporosis with your doctor. Most doctors will place you on calcium and vitamin D supplements if you're on chronic corticosteroids. Your doctor may also recommend taking them every other day.

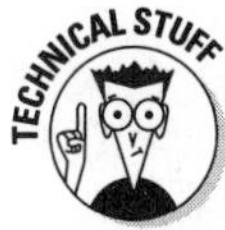

People on long-term moderate or high doses of corticosteroids may gain weight, develop hypertension or elevated blood sugars, and become prone to easy bruising. This condition is referred to as *iatrogenic* (a disease caused by medical treatment) Cushing's syndrome. These people are at most risk for bone loss.

Avoiding excess thyroid medication

Your thyroid is an important part of your body because it helps control your metabolism. Thyroid problems come in two varieties: *hypothyroid* (sometimes called Hashimoto's disease), or too little thyroid hormone being manufactured, and *hyperthyroid* (sometimes called Grave's disease), which is too much thyroid hormone. (If you want the complete lowdown on thyroid disease, check out *Thyroid For Dummies* by Alan L. Rubin, MD [Wiley].)

If your thyroid is underactive, you may gain weight, be tired all the time, feel cold, or have hair loss. If you have an overactive thyroid, you may lose weight, feel like your mind is racing, have difficulty sleeping, be jittery, and perspire more than usual.

Hyperthyroid hormone levels can increase your risk of developing osteoporosis. Hyperthyroid can result when your thyroid produces too much thyroid hormone or when you take more thyroid medication than you need to correct hypothyroidism.

A simple blood test ordered by your doctor can tell you whether or not the amount of medication you're taking is too much — or just enough.

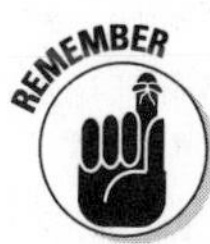

Calcium may interfere with absorption of your thyroid medication if the two are taken too close together. Your doctor may recommend taking your thyroid medicine in the morning and your calcium 12 hours later. You also need to avoid drinking calcium-fortified juices close to the time you take your thyroid medicine.

Taking medications to prevent seizures

Approximately one in ten people will have at least one seizure in their lifetime by age 75. There are different types of seizures caused by the malfunctioning of different parts of your brain; some seizure medications work better on one type of seizure than another. Some anti-epileptic drugs (AEDs) are more sedating than others, and many have been implicated in causing bone loss by interfering with your body's absorption of vitamin D.

Seizure medications may also interfere with female hormone levels such as estrogen and progesterone. Some AEDs suppress ovulation, which keeps estrogen levels from rising during the menstrual cycle. Lower estrogen levels means a greater chance of developing osteoporosis.

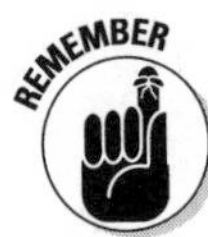

If you're on AEDs, make sure to have a bone density test done each year, and take at least 200 to 400 IU of vitamin D a day, along with at least 1,000 to 1,400 mg of calcium. Also be aware of a major risk of poorly controlled seizures: falling!

Other drugs associated with developing osteoporosis

A large number of drugs in addition to the ones in this section are associated with bone loss. Be aware that you may be at extra risk for osteoporosis if you're taking any of the following:

- **Vitamin A (in excess of 3,000 micrograms per day):** Excess vitamin A may cause too much bone to be reabsorbed. (See Chapter 11 about consuming too much vitamin A.)
- **Heparin, a blood thinner:** Researchers and doctors don't completely understand the connection between osteoporosis and heparin, but long-term therapy (more than four or five months) and doses of 15,000 IU or more increase the risk of osteoporosis. Heparin may increase the number of osteoclasts in bone. (See Chapter 2 for more on osteoclasts.)
- **Drugs that lower estrogen and testosterone:** Any drug that lowers your estrogen level increases your risk of developing osteoporosis because bone loss increases when estrogen levels are low. For example, Lupron (leuprolide acetate) is an anti-estrogen medicine that is used for women with endometriosis and also for certain cancers in men, such as prostate cancer. This drug lowers your estrogen level.

- **Medications that attack the virus that causes AIDS:** Anti-HIV drugs may increase your chance of osteoporosis by raising cholesterol levels and interfering with the way the body manufactures and uses fat.

How Gastrointestinal Problems Can Affect Your Bones

Your bones are dependent on what your digestive system absorbs, so anything that interferes with your absorption of calcium and vitamin D can weaken your bones. Diseases that wreak havoc with your insides can also wreak havoc with your bones. Eating well is important for development of strong bones (see Chapter 5 for more about nutrition and osteoporosis), but eating well won't help your bones if your intestines aren't absorbing the good stuff.

Vitamin D deficiency from inadequate nutrition might be more common that originally thought. In one recent study, 45 percent of hospitalized patients in Boston were vitamin D deficient. One cause of vitamin D deficiency is gastrointestinal diseases, which weren't looked for in those cases. See Chapter 11 for more information on vitamin D deficiency and its treatments.

Inflammatory bowel disease

If you have a chronic intestinal problem, such as ulcerative colitis or Crohn's disease, your risk for developing osteoporosis is threefold:

- The part of your intestine that absorbs vitamin D may be damaged by inflammation, and therefore you become vitamin D deficient.
- You may have had surgery, which removed the part of your intestine that absorbs vitamin D.
- You may be taking medications, such as corticosteroids, which increase bone loss. (See the section "Why corticosteroids can thin bones" earlier in this chapter.)

Your bone density may improve if your disease is in remission and you're no longer taking corticosteroids.

Bone loss after stomach surgery

New studies have shown that many people lose bone faster than they can replace it in the months following bariatric surgery to induce weight loss. Those people who lose the most weight and those people who lose weight quickly are most at risk, with up to an 8 percent drop in bone density six months after surgery. This loss may be the result of less efficient absorption of calcium, to the weight loss itself, or to the fact that vitamin D isn't adequately absorbed if part of the small intestine is removed.

Some people develop *osteomalacia,* a defect in the body's ability to mineralize bone, after stomach surgery. Osteomalacia (see Chapter 1 for more info) is considered to be "adult rickets" and results in many fractures in unusual places (ribs, pelvic bones, and shoulder blades).

Differentiating between osteoporosis and osteomalacia is important because treatment may differ. Your doctor can perform a bone biopsy to determine which condition is present. Bone biopsies are simple procedures to perform, but pathologists with special training in bone diseases need to interpret the results so that you receive the proper treatment.

Celiac disease and bone loss

As many as 1 in 250 men and women have an inherited disease called *celiac disease,* or nontropical sprue. People with celiac disease don't absorb adequate nutrients through the small intestine because their intestinal lining is damaged by eaten gluten, which is found in wheat.

Severe celiac disease can be associated with marked deficiency of vitamin D and numerous fractures. Patients without obvious causes of osteoporosis need to be screened for celiac disease because it's fairly common. Your doctor can diagnose celiac disease with a combination of history, blood tests, and intestinal biopsies. All untreated patients need to have frequent bone density testing and vitamin D measurements.

Noting Other Diseases Associated with Osteoporosis

Many different diseases can increase your risk of developing osteoporosis. In many cases the medicine you take, such as corticosteroids, to treat the disease increases your risk. In other cases the disease itself can cause bone loss.

Some other diseases associated with increased risk of osteoporosis are

- **Chronic kidney disease:** Kidney disease raises the amount of phosphate, a mineral that binds to calcium to maintain healthy bones, in the blood. The extra phosphate circulates in the blood looking for calcium to bind with, and will take calcium from your bones if necessary to attach to the phosphate, depleting your calcium stores.

  Some people with chronic kidney disease who are on dialysis develop a severe bone disorder known as *renal osteodystrophy.* Your kidneys are critical in the metabolism of vitamin D. When your kidneys start to fail, you become deficient in certain important active forms of vitamin D. Technically this condition isn't osteoporosis. A bone biopsy in this situation would reveal secondary hyperparathyroidism. Nonetheless, if you suffered from renal osteodystrophy, you could develop many fractures. A great deal of progress has been made in recent years in prevention and treatment of this disorder. Careful regulation of phosphorus levels and new forms of vitamin D supplementation have greatly reduced the incidence of this complex disorder.

- **Cirrhosis of the liver:** Many factors associated with liver failure can affect bone metabolism, such as the accumulation of toxins related to the ineffectiveness of the damaged liver to filter them out.
- **Ehler-Danlos syndrome:** This hereditary disease affects connective tissue and is associated with decreased bone density and hypermobility of joints.
- **Hypercalciuria:** People with hypercalciuria lose too much calcium through their urine, often in the form of calcium kidney stones. Your doctor might look for this problem by collecting your urine for 24 hours and measuring the amount of calcium in the urine.
- **Juvenile rheumatoid arthritis** and **rheumatoid arthritis:** People with rheumatoid arthritis are twice as likely to develop osteoporosis as the general population; the risk is even higher among rheumatoid arthritis patients who take corticosteroids.
- **Multiple myeloma:** This is a cancer of blood cells that results in bone tumors. Patients with multiple myeloma have abnormal plasma cells in their bone marrow. These cells make substances known as *cytokines* that stimulate osteoclasts and

inhibit osteoblasts, thus weakening the bone. (See Chapter 2 for the lowdown on osteoblasts and osteoclasts.)

- **Osteogenesis imperfecta (OI):** Several types of OI exist. Most are inherited and cause very brittle bones and fractures in childhood. OI is due to defects in the production of *collagen,* an important protein in the maintenance of bone strength. (See Chapter 4 for more information on osteoporosis in children.)
- **Overactive parathyroid gland:** An overactive parathyroid results in a rise in blood calcium levels, causing mental confusion, kidney damage, dehydration, nausea, and vomiting. (See Chapter 2 for more about hyperactive parathyroid glands.)
- **Overactive thyroid gland:** It negatively affects bone mineral density. (See "Avoiding excess thyroid medication" earlier in this chapter for more information.)

The problem is that doctors and researchers don't thoroughly understand the mechanism in these various diseases. For example, in people with Ehler-Danlos, the link could be genetic.

Reducing the Risks of Getting Osteoporosis

Osteoporosis isn't just an inevitable part of getting older or a disease that only women get. It's a complicated disease that can have many causes, and it's also a disease you can prevent by being proactive about your health.

Women do develop osteoporosis more frequently than men. So, given the fact that if you were born a woman, you're most likely going to stay one your whole life, what can you do to reduce your risk of osteoporosis? Be aware that osteoporosis is more common in women and start early to prevent it. Use these helpful tips and keep osteoporosis at bay:

- **Eat well from an early age if possible.** If you're already "over the hill," start eating well now, making sure you get at least 1,200 to 1,500 mg of calcium daily and 800 IU of vitamin D. Take supplements if necessary, and medications as ordered by your doctor. (See Chapter 5 for more on nutrition and Chapter 11 for more on supplements.)
- **Exercise, exercise, exercise!** It helps you build more bone mass and protects what you already have. (See Chapter 6 for more on the benefits of exercise at any age.)

- **Don't smoke!** If you already are smoking, do whatever you can do to stop or least reduce the amount you smoke.
- **Limit your daily alcohol intake.** Have no more than one to two alcoholic drinks each day.
- **Take medications your doctor prescribes.** Studies have shown that up to half of all prescriptions written by doctors aren't filled or aren't taken properly. (See Chapter 10 for more on medications that fight osteoporosis.)
- **Keep other health problems closely monitored.** If you have other health problems, such as the ones listed in "Noting Other Diseases Associated with Osteoporosis," earlier in this section, make sure you're especially diligent about your diet, exercise, and medication routines.
- **Know your family history.** If osteoporosis runs in your family, start working on changing history by changing your diet and habits.

Lost in space: Astronauts and bone loss

Astronauts are at risk for osteoporosis because of their prolonged weightlessness. (Bet you never really gave that much thought, did you?) People who are confined to bed for long periods of time also have accelerated bone loss, perhaps because of the same mechanism: You need gravity for strong bones!

Chapter 4

Men and Kids Get Osteoporosis, Too

In This Chapter

- Examining who else gets osteoporosis (besides women)
- Diagnosing and treating osteoporosis in men
- Understanding adolescents and osteoporosis
- Realizing kids can get osteoporosis

Until recently, the emphasis on diagnosing and treating osteoporosis has been mainly on women. However, men also get osteoporosis, and in fairly significant numbers. The misconception that they don't can cause delays in their diagnosis and treatment. Adolescents and children can also have osteoporosis or a related bone disease.

In this chapter, we look at the osteoporosis patients who don't get a lot of attention in the media: men, teens, and children.

Taking a Closer Look at Who Else Gets Osteoporosis

Although many osteoporosis sufferers are women, men and children can also have osteoporosis (see "Yes, Little Kids Can Have Osteoporosis" later in this chapter for more on children). In fact, 20 million men in the United States have osteoporosis, and one in four men older than age 50 will have an osteoporotic-related fracture in his lifetime. This chapter goes into more depth on how osteoporosis affects men, teens, and children, but first check out these interesting facts that may surprise you:

- Because men don't go through menopause, with its sudden drop in hormone levels, their onset of osteoporosis is later. But by age 65, men are losing bone at the same rate as women.
- Men of any race can have osteoporosis. Between 3 and 7 percent of men age 50 and older have osteoporosis, and between 19 and 35 percent have low bone mass. Men of Caucasian and Asian backgrounds are more likely to have low bone mass than African Americans or Hispanics.
- Juvenile osteoporosis is rare, and most often associated with other health conditions, although a form of osteoporosis called idiopathic juvenile osteoporosis (IJO) has been documented in a small number (less than 100) of previously healthy children just before the onset of adolescence. (See the sidebar "A rarity: Idiopathic juvenile osteoporosis" later in this chapter.)
- Girls who take being thin and athletic to an extreme may develop a syndrome called the female athlete triad, which can have permanent devastating effects on bone. (Check out the "The female athlete triad" section later in this chapter for more info.)

Focusing on Osteoporosis in Men

Although most of the research has focused on women with osteoporosis, researchers are slowly starting to place more emphasis on understanding when and why men develop osteoporosis.

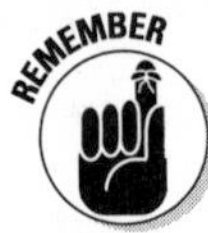

Men generally start adulthood with larger, heavier bones than women, and have a higher peak bone mass. But between 15 to 25 percent of all men will develop osteoporosis, and after age 50, 6 percent will fracture their hip. Table 4-1 shows the relationship of hip fractures in men and women more clearly:

Table 4-1 Comparing Osteoporosis-Related Hip Fractures in Men and Women

Factor	*Men*	*Women*
Peak bone mass	10 to 12 percent higher than women	
Lifetime risk of hip fracture	6 percent	17 percent

Factor	*Men*	*Women*
Mortality from hip fracture	31 percent	17 percent
Sex distribution of hip fractures worldwide	30 percent	70 percent
U.S. incidence of hip fracture at age 65	4 to 5 per 1000	8 to 10 per 1000

Osteoporosis begins to affect men about ten years later than it affects women. And because both men and women are living longer, researchers and doctors anticipate more people will have hip fractures in the future. In fact, by the year 2050, researchers project that men will have one half of all hip fractures in the United States.

By the age of 86, the incidence of hip fracture in men is *equal* to the incidence in women, meaning that by age 86, osteoporosis isn't a "women's disease" in any way.

Because osteoporosis apparently becomes an equal opportunity disease as you age, you may be curious as to when men should start having bone mineral density scans. All men older than 70 need a baseline scan, as well as men under age 70 who have risk factors, such as long-term corticosteroid use or use of drugs to treat prostate cancer. (See Chapter 9 for more information on baseline scans, and check out the next section for more on risk factors in men.)

Seeking answers in the "Mr. OS" study

A seven-year study begun in 1999 by the NIH National Institute of Arthritis and Musculoskeletal and Skin Diseases (NIAMS), along with the National Institute on Aging and National Cancer Institute is following 5,700 men older than age 65. The study, called "Mr. OS," is looking at men's risk factors for osteoporosis and how osteoporosis affects men specifically. Knowledge of the diseases and conditions that can affect bone mass can help to prevent men as well as women from reaching the point of fracture before diagnosis.

One part of the study is looking at the possible relationship between high bone mass and prostate cancer. This increased risk may be related to levels of hormones, such as testosterone, which protect bone. Other findings that are being examined in the study include the following:

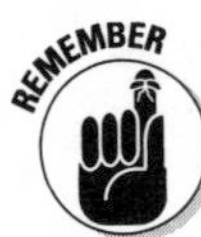

- Although men sustain hip fractures less frequently than women, their mortality rate one year after hip fracture is two to three times higher than for women.
- Risk factors for developing osteoporosis appear to be the same in men as in women:
  - **Alcohol abuse:** Alcohol abuse increases bone loss. Approximately 25 to 50 percent of men seeking treatment for alcohol abuse have low bone mass.
  - **Inadequate calcium and vitamin D intake:** Men older than 50 must consume 1,200 mg of calcium and 400 to 800 International Units (IU) of vitamin D daily.
  - **Lack of exercise:** Men, like women, need to do weight-bearing exercise 20 to 30 minutes a day three days a week to build bone strength. (See Chapter 6 for more on exercise.)
  - **Low hormone levels:** Up to 30 percent of men with osteoporosis have low testosterone levels and may need hormone replacement. In one study, one-third of men older than 70 with a fracture were *hypogonadal,* or suffering from low testosterone levels. *Hypogonadism* is often underdiagnosed in men because there's no obvious precipitating event. In women, when estrogen levels drop and menopause begins, their menses stops and hot flashes start. But in men, during andropause, falling testosterone levels may not be detected. Hence, *andropause* (male menopause) may be subtler than menopause in women, because signs of andropause might just be attributed to aging, such as lack of sex drive or difficulty maintaining an erection.
  - **Prostate cancer:** Chemotherapy to treat prostate cancer and other malignancies may also lower testosterone levels.
  - **Smoking:** Men who smoke are two to three times as likely to fracture vertebrae as nonsmokers.
  - **Use of corticosteroids for diseases, such as asthma:** Men who have osteoporosis are more likely than women to develop the disease because of another medical condition or because of medication they take, such as

corticosteroids. Use of corticosteroids accounts for between 15 to 20 percent of osteoporosis in men. Men taking these drugs need to maintain an adequate calcium intake, have their testosterone levels checked, and may need to take antiresorptive medications (see Chapter 11 for more on osteoporosis medications).

Table 4-2 compares the risk factors for men developing osteoporosis and divides them into high, medium, and less common risks.

Table 4-2 Comparing the Risk Factors for Men Developing Osteoporosis

High Risk Factors	***Medium Risk Factors***	***Less Common Causes***
Corticosteroid use of 5 mgm or more per day times six months	Alcohol abuse	Cushing disease
Hyperparathyroidism	Anticonvulsant drugs	Gastric resection
Hypogonadism	Family history of osteoporosis	Low body weight
Nontraumatic fracture of hip, vertebrae, or wrist	Hypo- or hyperthyroidism	Liver or kidney disease
Osteopenia seen on X-ray	Multiple myeloma or lymphoma	
	Rheumatoid or inflammatory arthritis	
	Risk of falling due to unstable gait, dementia, or stroke	

Treating men with osteoporosis

Because osteoporosis is recognized in men less often than in women, fewer men are put on medication to reduce the risk of osteoporosis until the damage has already been done. However, studies are beginning to show that the same drugs successfully used to treat women with osteoporosis also help men (see Chapter 10 for medications used to treat osteoporosis). The major difference in treatment in men and women is that hormone replacement differs.

In 2001, the FDA approved use of alendronate (Fosamax) in treatment of osteoporosis in men. Before this point in time, few studies had been done exclusively in men. Just after that, Forteo was approved to treat osteoporosis in both men and women.

Because many men who develop osteoporosis have low levels of testosterone, which drops gradually as they age, they may need to take testosterone supplements. *Androgens,* or male sex hormones, such as testosterone, stimulate bone formation. Doctors may prescribe testosterone in the form of injections, patches, or gel to raise the testosterone to normal levels.

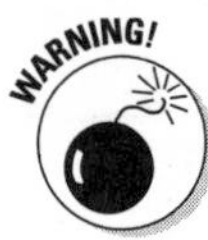

Although testosterone is effective in reducing calcium loss and helping to maintain bone density, it isn't without side effects. Men with prostate cancer shouldn't take testosterone, because prostate tumors may grow larger with added testosterone. Other potential side effects of testosterone therapy include enlargement of the breasts, swelling of hands and feet, and erectile dysfunction.

Researchers are studying new ways to give testosterone, such as patches, injections, under the tongue, or gel, that may bypass the liver. When the drug doesn't pass through the liver, the chances of liver damage are greatly reduced. Bypassing the liver can also result in more of the drug being available for absorption.

Don't take testosterone replacement therapy if you have

- Breast cancer (men can get that too)
- Liver disease
- *Polycythemia* (an abnormal increase in the number of red blood cells)
- Prostate cancer

Avoid DHEA (a steroid hormone that decreases with age and is often sold as a "rejuvenation" drug in health food stores) supplements if you're taking testosterone, because the combination of the two may be dangerous.

Researchers are also working to develop designer androgens that might have the desired bony effects without increasing the risk of prostate cancer.

Prostate cancer and osteoporosis

Some evidence suggests that men who have prostate cancer and are receiving androgen-deprivation therapy are at increased risk for osteoporosis. Androgen-deprivation therapy focuses on decreasing the level of testosterone in men with prostate cancer, because testosterone may encourage growth of the cancerous cells. Around 40 percent of men with prostate cancer receive antihormone therapy as part of their treatment.

One large study showed that men who had received nine or more doses of hormone therapy were 45 percent more likely to sustain a bone fracture and had a 66 percent higher chance of needing hospitalization after a fracture. Another study showed that five years after treatment, slightly more than 19 percent of men had a fracture, compared to 12.6 percent of men who hadn't had any antihormone therapy.

Taking drugs to fight osteoporosis called *bisphosphonates* (see Chapter 10 for more on bisphosphonates) may reduce the risk of bone loss and consequent fractures in men taking antihormone drugs, such as leuprolide acetate (Lupron). If you're taking an antihormone drug, ask your doctor about taking bisphosphonates to help offset bone loss.

Focusing on prevention and treatment

Outside of the use of testosterone in men, prevention and treatment of osteoporosis in men and women is similar. Whether you're male or female, the best way to treat osteoporosis is to prevent it from happening, by eating well, exercising, and by not smoking or drinking alcohol excessively. (See Chapter 3, which covers all the prevention measures you can take to avoid osteoporosis.)

The older you get

Nobody ever said getting older was a picnic. When it comes to prostate cancer, the most common cancer found in American men, outside of skin cancer, age is definitely against you. Although men have a one in six lifetime risk of developing prostate cancer, the risk increases dramatically, to one in two, if you make it to age 80. The good news is that prostate cancer is a slow-growing cancer, and has a high cure rate depending on whether or not the cancer has begun to spread to other organs before it's discovered. The best way to beat prostate cancer is to catch it early by having a regular blood test screening called prostate specific antigen (PSA) or a digital rectal exam.

If you already have osteoporosis, check out Chapter 10 for effective medication treatments.

Why Too Thin Is Bad for Bones — Especially in Teens

You may remember the teenage angst of feeling "too fat," even when your weight barely touched the 100-pound mark. Teens today are as acutely aware of their weight, and many, if not most, teenage girls want to be thin. Unfortunately, the desire to be thin can lead to behaviors that can have disastrous consequences for bones down the road.

Because the teen years are so important in building the bone mass that you draw from for the rest of your life, behaviors aimed at staying thin, such as smoking and excessive dieting, will result in bone loss that can never be regained, even if you change behaviors as an adult.

For example, some teenage girls see smoking cigarettes as a way to curb their weight. One Japanese study showed teens that were concerned about their weight were four times more likely to start smoking. In fact, nearly 30 percent of American teenage girls are regular smokers.

Dieting and bone loss

Avoiding the "it's in to be thin" emphasis today is difficult, especially if you're young and impressionable. Being severely underweight can have devastating consequences to bone, especially if there is an associated eating disorder, such as anorexia and bulimia.

The American Psychiatric Society defines anorexia nervosa and bulimia nervosa in the following way:

Anorexia nervosa is

- A refusal to maintain weight that's over the lowest weight considered normal for age and height
- An intense fear of gaining weight or becoming fat, even though underweight
- A distorted body image
- In women, three consecutive missed menstrual periods without pregnancy

Finding out a bit more about anorexia

The following important tidbits are important to know about anorexia nervosa and how it can affect bone development:

- Anorexia nervosa is a psychological disease that has physical consequences lasting all through life. Around 1 out of 100 adolescents, 90 percent of whom are female, develops anorexia.
- Anorexia can cause bone loss in several ways. Girls with anorexia stop having menstrual periods because their estrogen levels fall too low due to a lack of body fat. Falling estrogen levels are a prime cause for a decrease in bone density.
- Anorexics generally don't consume an adequate amount of calories, which results in less bone formation during adolescence, a time when up to half of peak bone density is being achieved. In addition, anorexics often have a high level of a glucocorticoid called cortisol, which contributes to bone loss.
- Teens with anorexia have been found to have spinal density 25 percent less than that of healthy teens, and up to two-thirds of anorectics have bone density more than two standard deviations below the normal on a DXA scan, a test done to determine your bone density. (See Chapter 9 for more about DXA scans and how to interpret them.)

Doctors and counselors direct treatment of anorexia at achieving weight gain. When an anorexic reaches 90 percent of her normal body weight, her period usually resumes. Estrogen therapy may also help. Studies have shown that bone lost during this time period isn't easily regained, and the increased risk of fracture may be permanent, even with treatment.

Meanwhile, *bulimia nervosa* is

- Recurrent episodes of *binge eating,* which means eating more than needed to satisfy hunger; (minimum average of two binge-eating episodes a week for at least three months)
- A feeling of lack of control over eating during the binges
- A regular use of one or more of the following to prevent weight gain:
  - Self-induced vomiting
  - Strict dieting or fasting
  - Use of laxatives or diuretics
  - Vigorous exercise
- A persistent over-concern with body shape and weight

Bulimics aren't always underweight; many maintain their weight within normal limits and don't experience the stopping of menstrual periods and bone loss that anorexics do.

The female athlete triad

The *female athlete triad* may sound like some sort of Olympic event, but it actually describes a serious result of eating disorders combined with too much exercise. Young athletes involved in sports, such as ballet, gymnastics, and figure skating, where keeping their weight low is important, often suffer from this condition.

What causes this condition? The combination of stringent dieting and excessive exercise results in a loss of menstrual periods, which lowers estrogen levels. The outcome? The athlete lacks the nutrients to grow strong bones and hormones to maintain bone, which causes osteoporosis at a young age, leading to stress fractures and weakened bones that can last a lifetime.

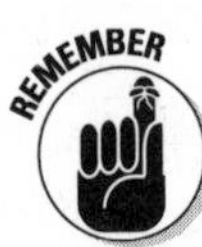

A young athlete may seem to be taking in a normal number of calories, but the amount eaten may be far below what she needs because of her greatly increased physical activity.

The female athlete triad isn't an uncommon problem. In fact, among female athletes, the syndrome may be present in as many as 50 percent or more of athletes. If you're a parent, grandparent, or close friend of a young athlete, watch for these signs to see if the child is taking training to a dangerous level:

- Loss of menstrual periods for three months in a row
- Preoccupation with eating and/or using diet pills, laxatives, or diuretics
- Frequent visits to the bathroom immediately after eating
- Menstruation not begun by age 16
- Always wearing baggy sweatshirts and pants so weight loss isn't evident

Girls with the female athlete triad may be put on hormone replacement therapy to supply necessary hormones. They also need to be under a physician's care.

If you're the relative, coach, or friend of a young athlete, how can you help them avoid the trap of the female athlete triad? Follow these three simple steps:

1. **Don't emphasize winning as the most important thing.**

   The benefits of sports are many, and although winning is great, don't seek it at the price of permanent health problems.

2. **Be aware.**

   Watch for the signs that your athlete is taking diet and exercise to an extreme, and don't wait until you notice everything is out of hand before doing something about it.

3. **Take action.**

   Don't bury your head in the sand when you see signs. Don't assume that just talking to your athlete will fix the problem. Enlist the help of your doctor and the coach.

Yes, Little Kids Can Have Osteoporosis

Even though osteoporosis is rarer in children, it can occur. But some diseases, such as rickets, osteogenesis imperfecta, and the very rare idiopathic juvenile osteoporosis (IOA), can also cause osteoporosis or bone loss in children. And some medical treatments, such as corticosteroids to treat asthma, can also lead to osteoporosis. This section examines these conditions in more detail.

Rickets: A real risk for bone loss

You may think of rickets as a disease of the past, and to some extent you're correct. Rickets, a vitamin D deficiency, was much more common before the early 1920s, before milk was fortified with vitamin D and rickets greatly decreased.

But rickets is still around, although it's not a common disease. In adults, rickets is known as *osteomalacia* (see Chapter 1 for more on osteomalacia). Rickets and osteomalacia both have the same causes and effects.

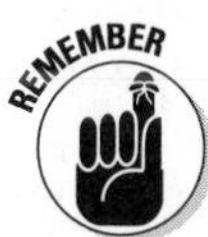

Some of the symptoms of rickets are

- Bone fractures
- Bone pain
- Fever, restlessness, and weakness

- Growing wings and jumping from grass blade to grass blade (Wait, ignore that. That's from *Crickets For Dummies.*)
- Muscle cramps
- Short stature
- Skeletal deformities such as bowlegs, pigeon breast, spine curvatures, or odd-shaped skull
- Soft teeth

Rickets is a childhood metabolic disease that causes an imbalance between bone breakdown and remodeling. This imbalance can happen because the child isn't taking in enough vitamin D, or because an intestinal disease, such as celiac disease (or sprue), is blocking the absorption of vitamin D.

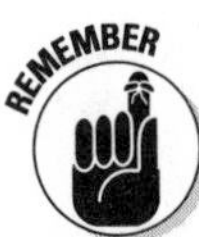

Vitamin D is available from two sources: sunlight and food. In industrial areas, pollution may block sunlight. In cold areas, sunlight may be limited during the winter. People with dark skin absorb less sunlight and are more prone to vitamin D deficiency.

Newborns sometimes are vitamin D deficient because their breastfeeding mothers are. Breast milk normally doesn't contain adequate amounts of vitamin D, but the amount can be increased if mom takes vitamin D supplements. Breastfed babies can also take supplements.

Sometimes children with special diets can develop rickets. For example, a child allergic to milk and dairy products or a vegetarian child who avoids milk products needs vitamin D supplementation to avoid rickets. Consult with your doctor about the appropriate amounts, depending on your child's age.

A hereditary inability of the kidneys to retain phosphate or a kidney disorder that causes acidosis can cause rickets. Liver disorders can also cause problems with vitamin D absorption or metabolism.

Osteogenesis imperfecta (OI)

Osteogenesis imperfecta (OI) is a genetic bone disease usually inherited from a parent. Occasionally, OI occurs as a spontaneous mutation with no family history. A parent with OI has a 50 percent chance of passing the gene on to a child.

A rarity: Idiopathic juvenile osteoporosis (IJO)

Idiopathic juvenile osteoporosis (IJO) is a rare disease, with less than 100 cases reported, and occurs in previously healthy children between the ages of 4 and 16. Most of the time, the disease goes into spontaneous remission within two to four years.

Children with IJO may complain of pain in their back, hips, and feet, and may have trouble walking. Their DXA scans may show low bone density, and X-rays will reveal fractures of weight-bearing bone or collapsed vertebrae.

Treatment of IJO is aimed at protecting bones from fracture until remission occurs, through physical therapy and reduced activity. Doctors generally don't use medications unless the disease is severe and not resolving spontaneously.

Damage from IJO can result in permanent collapse of the rib cage or scoliosis, but often the disease leaves no permanent disability. Growth may be hindered during the active phase of the disease, but normal growth usually resumes in remission. Most children experience complete recovery with no later recurrence.

People with OI are missing a protein called *type I collagen.* This protein helps make up bone, ligaments, teeth, and the white outer part of the eyeball, the *sclera.* The lack of type I collagen creates fragile bone that fractures easily, although it heals at a normal rate.

OI can range from mild to severe, and anywhere between 20,000 and 50,000 people in the United States have OI. Some individuals with OI have distinctive features: They're shorter than average. They have a blue, gray, or purple tint to the whites of their eyes. Some have hearing loss.

Someone with OI may have anywhere from ten fractures to hundreds in their lifetime. Some fractures may need surgical treatment. For example, metal rods may need to be inserted into the long bones of the arms and legs. Spinal fusion may be necessary to limit scoliosis. The rate of fracture often declines as OI children become adults, but may increase again as women enter menopause.

Doctors aim treatment at maximizing function, minimizing disability, and maintaining overall health and independence. Doctors may prescribe an injectable bisphosphonate drug, pamidronate (Aredia), to strengthen bones and reduce fractures.

If your child or grandchild suffers from IO, take extra care when handling him. (Don't avoid touching your child. Give him or her plenty of hugs and kisses — just be gentle.) Casts are probably going to be a way of life for your child, so make sure the car seat and stroller you buy are big enough to accommodate them.

Corticosteroids and osteoporosis in children

The use of corticosteroids for inflammatory diseases, such as asthma, in children is one of the biggest childhood risks for developing osteoporosis.

Most children who develop corticosteroid-induced osteoporosis are taking oral steroids. Although researchers and doctors haven't ruled out high-dose inhaled steroids as a possible cause of osteoporosis, studies haven't been conclusive (see "Substituting inhaled corticosteroids" later in this section). If your child is likely to be on oral corticosteroids long term, ask your doctor to conduct a baseline bone densitometry to monitor any changes (check out Chapter 9 for more on baseline testing).

One study by the National Jewish Medical and Research Center of 400 asthmatic children on daily oral corticosteroids made the following conclusions:

- Daily doses of 10 mg of prednisone can cause bone loss.
- Thirty to 50 percent of children will have bone loss.
- Bone loss in children will be mainly in the vertebrae and *radius* (forearm).
- Bone loss won't have any symptoms until a fracture occurs.
- Bone densitometry starting at age 5 is essential in high-risk children.
- Bone loss is most common in children taking a daily dose of 20 mg or more of a corticosteroid. Short "bursts" or occasional corticosteroid use doesn't appear to cause bone loss.

Substituting inhaled corticosteroids

Although studies measuring possible bone loss in children who have used inhaled corticosteroids have been inconclusive, some preliminary results show less chance of bone loss and osteoporosis if the children use inhaled corticosteroids rather than oral ones.

Studies have shown some conflicting information, however. In 2001, studies in young women showed that inhaled corticosteroids to treat asthma resulted in loss of bone density. Eight puffs daily had the greatest effect. Then in 2003, further data appeared in the literature that showed that inhaled corticosteroids in children didn't seem to affect bone. These preliminary results are great news, but need to be viewed with caution, because there is conflicting information.

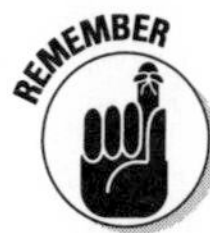

Several studies in adult asthmatics have shown decreases in *osteocalcin,* a protein made by bone forming osteoclasts, in inhaled corticosteroid users, so inhaled corticosteroids could possibly be damaging, although not to the same extent as oral doses.

With chronic disease requiring the daily use of corticosteroids, the best advice is to start with the smallest dose that gives good effect, start with inhaled corticosteroids rather than oral doses if possible, and monitor bone closely. Keep the number of puffs used daily to a minimum. Inhaled corticosteroids for asthma are critically important in treating this potentially life-threatening and lung-damaging problem.

Treating corticosteroid-induced osteoporosis

Like it or not, some children need to be on daily doses of oral corticosteroids. The treatment goal is to minimize bone damage, even if it can't be avoided completely. If your child takes oral corticosteroids, ask your doctor to start with the lowest effective dose to treat, instead of pulling out the big guns from the start.

Children on corticosteroids must maintain an adequate calcium and vitamin D intake. This amount may be higher than the normal recommended daily allowance, which for calcium is 400 mg for infants aged 0 to 6 months, 800 mg for children 1 to 10, and 1,200 mg for adolescents and young adults 11 to 25. Children on corticosteroids need to have 1,000 to 1,500 mg of calcium daily, and 400 to 800 IU of vitamin D.

Furthermore, keep your child exercising, even if you and your doctor have to modify the exercise program for your child's limitations. Maintaining weight-bearing activities stimulates bone mass.

Have a baseline bone densitometry test done so your doctor can watch for any changes. Your doctor may also want to monitor 24-hour urinary calcium, phosphorus, and *creatinine* (a waste product that can help measure kidney function) levels to check for mineral loss. Taking blood tests for *osteocalcin,* which helps measure bone turnover, may also be helpful.

Part II
Keeping Your Bones Healthy

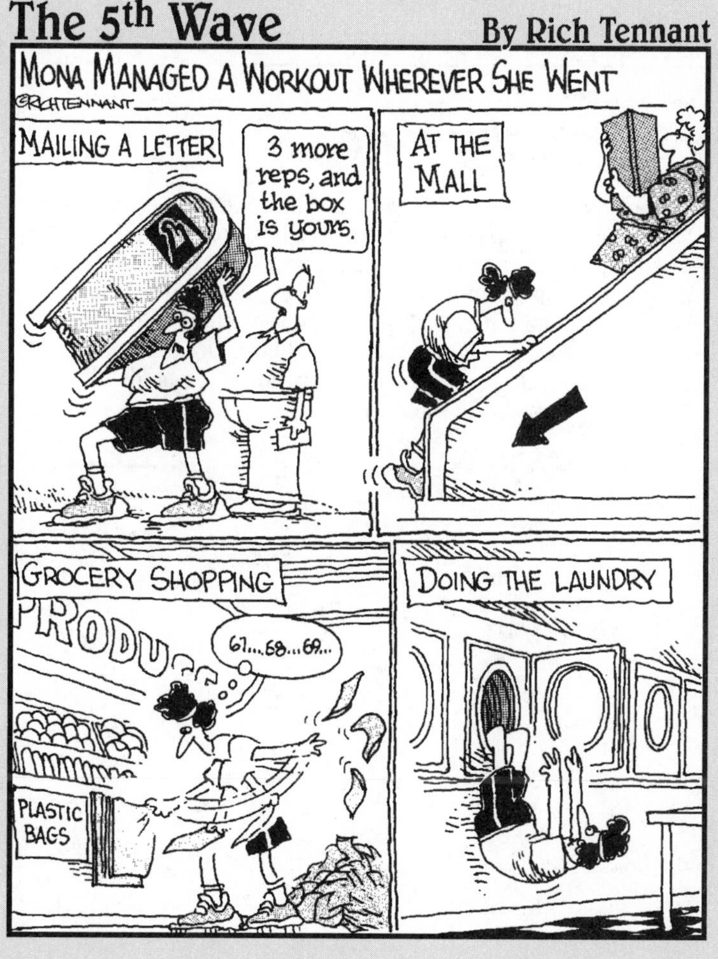

In this part . . .

Bones need love and care to reach their potential. In this part, we educate you on what bones need to grow big and strong and stay that way. Worried about not getting enough calcium to build strong bones because you're not a milk drinker? We have great suggestions for increasing calcium without a single glass. Dreading exercise? We include some easy-to-do-at-home ideas for increasing your bone strength.

Chapter 5

Eating Right for Good Bones

In This Chapter

- Consuming enough calcium and vitamin D
- Adding up other minerals
- Stopping the saltshaker shake
- Comparing high and low protein diets
- Understanding alcohol's effect on your bones
- Calming the caffeine buzz
- Balancing weighty issues

Is it true that "you are what you eat?" When it comes to building bones, which are strong enough to last a lifetime, the answer is a resounding *yes!*

You not only are what you eat today, but you're also what you ate three weeks ago, three months, three years, and so on. Your bones today are strong because of the calcium you ate during your formative years, up to age 30 or so. If you ate poorly, didn't exercise, and smoked and drank too much alcohol, your bones are going to pay the price — and not just today, but years from now as well.

The bone mass you build by your mid-20s or 30s is the best you'll ever have. After that, all you can do is maintain what you have; you can't build any more. The amount of bone gained during adolescence should equal the amount lost during the rest of your adult lifetime. If you don't build enough bone in adolescence, you'll have too little to "draw from" during the later part of your life.

Although heredity and certain unchangeable factors, such as race, body build, and gender, play a large part in determining your peak bone mass, up to 50 percent can be attributed to lifestyle behaviors. And eating is certainly a lifestyle behavior.

In this chapter, we tell you what to eat today to maintain strong bones and how to plan a lifelong diet to keep what you've built. If you're just starting to think about your bones after a lifetime of ignoring them, we can recommend some food strategies.

Getting Enough Calcium in Your Diet

When you hear the words "healthy bones," your first thought may be "I need to consume more food rich in calcium." For many of you this statement is true, because most Americans don't get enough calcium from their diets. As convenient as supplements may be, the calcium that's best absorbed is the calcium you get from your diet.

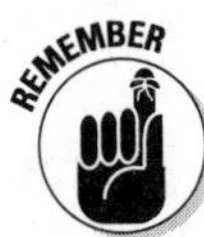

Calcium is only one of the minerals responsible for maintaining your bones, but it's a very important one, and one in which as many as 35 percent of Americans are deficient. (See Chapter 2 for more on the relationship between calcium and your bones.)

Most of the time, your body keeps a steady amount of calcium. So when you don't have enough calcium in your diet, your bones get less than they need to maintain strength. Leaving your bones short of calcium may not kill you, at least not directly, but it does have a large negative effect on your life if it leads to osteoporotic fractures.

Because getting "enough" calcium is a nebulous term, we devise Table 5-1 to show you exactly how much calcium you need at different points in your life.

Table 5-1 Getting Enough Calcium at Every Age

Age	*Recommended Daily Calcium Intake in Milligrams*
0 to 6 months	210
7 to 12 months	270
1 to 3 years	500
4 to 8 years	800
9 to 18 years	1,300
19 to 50 years	1,000
Older than 50	1,200

You may be surprised to see that adults need more calcium than babies and young children because many people mistakenly believe that milk and other calcium-rich foods are mostly for babies and children. Although a good calcium intake at younger ages is important so that bones reach their maximum strength, a good calcium intake is just as important as you get older so that you can maintain the bone you already have.

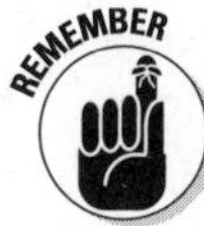

If you're a parent or grandparent, you can demonstrate what a good diet looks like by including ample amounts of calcium in your diet. You know that lecturing little ears about getting enough calcium and restricting foods that deplete calcium, such as soft drinks, likely falls upon deaf ears. Kids don't care what's going to happen to their bones in 30 years.

You need to make sure the choices your children and grandchildren are offered can build strong bones from a young age. And young adults must know that you can't let good habits slide just because you're no longer building bone mass. A common misconception is that after you achieve your maximum height, you can discontinue drinking milk. Not so fast!

The fact is children between the ages of 9 and 18 require the highest amount of calcium (1,300 mg per day). For postmenopausal women, the recommended dietary allowance (RDA) is 1,200 mg per day, which is only a 100 mg less! Most physicians recommend 1,500 mg of calcium daily if you're diagnosed with osteoporosis.

Hence stopping your good eating habits and assuming that you've done enough by eating well in your childhood and teens is a mistake. Studies show that you have to maintain your calcium intake for its positive effects on your bones to continue.

You probably know that dairy products are great sources of calcium. If you're not big on dairy, check out Chapter 15, which includes ten great alternatives to dairy products to reach your daily calcium levels. You can manage to keep up your calcium intake and never touch a single dairy product, but you'll have to add carefully.

Don't shut this book if you're thinking to yourself, "I hate milk, and I'm not going to drink milk, even if my bones start crumbling like potato chips." Don't be hasty — we also include tons of suggestions in this chapter about how you can get an adequate amount of calcium without ever opening a milk carton.

Milk matters!

You've probably seen the milk-mustachioed personalities featured in the "Got Milk?" ads. The campaign to increase milk consumption has also spawned T-shirts and, of course, parodies.

Why the emphasis on milk? Obviously, the "Got Milk?" campaign is designed to sell more milk. But the focus on milk as a good food is a wonderful thing. Milk consumption increased by 15 million gallons the first year the ads aired in California. So what's milk got that other dairy foods don't, besides a clever campaign? The answer is: more calcium.

A cup of calcium-fortified milk contains 420 mg of calcium, about a third of your daily requirement. It doesn't matter if it's 2 percent, skim, or whole milk; milk is the hands-down winner of the high calcium award. The commercial brought national attention to the fact that today's youth were consuming less milk and more soft drinks. For more on the "Got Milk?" campaign, visit its Web site at `www.whymilk.com`.

Table 5-2 shows that milk is an excellent source of calcium, but so are some other foods. (See Tables 5-2, 5-3, and 5-4.) And don't forget that milk is milk, even if you mix it into your mashed potatoes instead of chugging it from the carton.

Table 5-2 Dairy and Nondairy Sources for Calcium

Food Source	*Portion Size*	*Calcium in Milligrams*
Dairy Sources		
Cheese, hard	1 ounce	240
Cheese, processed	2 slices	265
Cottage cheese	¾ cup	120
Frozen yogurt	½ cup	100
Ice cream	½ cup	85
Milk, fortified	1 cup	420
Milk, whole, 2%. Skim, without added calcium	1 cup	300

Food Source	*Portion Size*	*Calcium in Milligrams*
Yogurt, low fat, plain	¾ cup	300
Yogurt, fruit bottom	¾ cup	250
Nondairy Drinks		
Calcium-fortified orange juice	1 cup	300
Fortified soymilk	1 cup	300 (not as well absorbed as cow's milk)

Table 5-3 Beans, Fruits, Grains, and Nuts

Food Source	*Portion Size*	*Calcium in Milligrams*
Beans and Bean Products		
Black turtle beans	½ cup	50
Navy beans	½ cup	60
Tofu, firm, made with calcium sulphate	3.5 ounces	125
Pinto beans, chickpeas	½ cup	40
White beans	½ cup	100
Fruits		
Dried figs	2 medium	54
Orange	1 medium	55
Grains		
Whole wheat flour	1 cup	40
Nuts and Seeds		
Almonds, dry roasted	¼ cup	95
Hazelnuts, brazil	¼ cup	55
Whole sesame seeds	1 tablespoon	90

Table 5-4 Other Sources of Dietary Calcium

Food	*Portion Size*	*Calcium in Milligrams*
Brown sugar	1 cup	180
Calcium-fortified bread and cereals	Varies	Varies — at least 100
Cornbread	2.5 inch square	80 to 90
Egg	1 medium	55
Molasses, blackstrap	1 tablespoon	170
Molasses, regular	1 tablespoon	40
Salmon, canned with bones	3 ounces	180
Sardines, canned	8 medium	370

As you can see, calcium isn't just for milk drinkers; you can find calcium in a number of other foods. Even fortified breads and cereals, depending on the manufacturer, typically contain at least 100 mg of calcium.

Living with lactose intolerance

Millions of people worldwide are *lactose intolerant,* meaning that they can't break down and use *lactose,* the main sugar found in milk and other dairy products. These people are deficient in the enzyme that breaks down lactose known as *lactase*. The symptoms include bloating, lower abdominal pains, and loose stools after drinking milk. As time goes by, people who are lactose intolerant often drink less milk to avoid the symptoms.

Lactose intolerance affects all races to some degree, although African Americans, Asian Americans, Hispanics, and Native Americans are affected more frequently than Caucasians. For example, some studies in the United States quote a 70 percent incidence in African Americans and a 15 percent incidence in Caucasians.

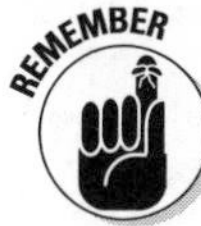

Lactose intolerant people are twice as likely to suffer from osteoporosis than people who aren't lactose intolerant. They have a higher rate of osteoporosis because they typically take in less calcium, or because they don't absorb calcium well.

You can take some easy steps to maintain your calcium intake if you're lactose intolerant by:

- **Drinking lactose-free milk, such as Lactaid.** In lactose-free milk, the lactose has been chemically removed.
- **Drinking soymilk.** We thank comedian Lewis Black for pointing out that soymilk is more appropriately referred to as "soy juice" because it doesn't come from a cow! Have you ever seen a soy cow before? Neither have we!
- **Trying Ultra Lactaid tablets.** Take one just before consuming any product with lactose. These tablets often aren't effective in people with severe deficiencies of the enzyme.
- **Checking our charts in this chapter for calcium contents of foods that don't contain lactose.** We provide plenty of alternatives, for example, oranges, almonds, and salmon. (A yummy spinach salad topped with orange slices, sliced almonds, and chunks of grilled salmon sounds good right now!)
- **Looking for calcium-fortified drinks, such as orange juice.** Make sure you know what you're getting by reading the label.
- **Eating yogurt with active cultures.** Yogurts with live active cultures contain bacteria that help digests lactose. (One cup of yogurt contains 5 grams of lactose.)
- **Chopping up some cheese.** Hard cheeses, such as cheddar and Swiss, have much of their lactose broken down during the production process. (Swiss cheese still has a gram of lactose.)

To get a better feel for how certain dairy foods compare to each other in terms of lactose content, check out Table 5-5.

Table 5-5 Lactose Content of Dairy Products

Dairy Food	*Grams of Lactose*
One ounce of Swiss cheese	1 gram
One cup of yogurt	5 grams
One cup of milk	11 grams
One cup of ice cream	12 grams

"Eat your leafy greens!"

Yes, your parents were right about eating your vegetables. Not only did your eating them keep peace at the dinner table, but they also helped build your future bones.

Nearly all vegetables contain some calcium. Generally speaking, if it's green and leafy, it's probably a good source of calcium. (Some vegetables, such as cauliflower, eggplant, and potatoes, only contain small amounts, around 10 mg per serving. Corn, beets, and mushrooms also register low on the calcium scale.) You also have to keep in mind how the calcium intake changes when you cook your vegetables (see Table 5-6).

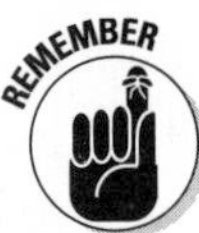

Some vegetables contain calcium that is more easily absorbed than others. The calcium in spinach, for example, isn't absorbed as well as the calcium in broccoli or kale, because spinach contains oxalic acid, which binds calcium.

Table 5-6 Calcium Amounts Found in Vegetables (Cooked)

Vegetable	*Amount*	*Percentage Daily Allowance of Calcium*
Broccoli	½ cup	35
Chinese cabbage	½ cup	75
Kale	½ cup	50
Mustard greens	½ cup	50
Okra	½ cup	75
Rutabaga	½ cup	40
Spinach	½ cup	75
Turnip greens	½ cup	95

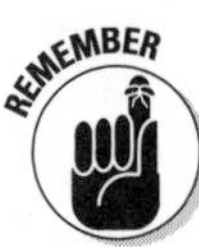

Another reason to eat your leafy greens: Recent studies have shown that a daily intake of three to five serving of fruits and vegetables daily can increase your calcium levels not only because they contain calcium, but also because their *acidity*, or *alkalinity*, increases the calcium that's able to be absorbed from them (see the "Looking at the acid test" sidebar later in this chapter).

Reading the labels: How much calcium is in it?

You can find nutritional labels (check out Figure 5-1) on almost everything these days. You can barely pick up anything at the grocery store that doesn't have a label with nutritional contents listed on it — like you really wanted to know that a corn muffin contains 500 calories!

Serving Size 1 cup (240 ml)

Calories 150 **Calories from Fat** 70

	Amount Per Serving	% Daily Value
Total Fat	8g	12%
Saturated Fat	5g	25%
Cholesterol	35mg	11%
Total Carbohydrate	12g	4%
Dietary Fiber	0g	0%
Sugars	12g	
Protein	8g	
Vitamin A		6%
Vitamin C		2%
Calcium		30%
Vitamin D		25%

Figure 5-1: A nutritional label from fortified whole milk.

When it comes to figuring out calcium amounts, the label makers have made it a bit more difficult by putting down a percentage, rather than an amount in milligrams. You can easily figure it out though.

If a label says that one serving contains 20 percent of the daily value, just multiply 20 by 10 and you've got the milligrams of calcium. So 20 percent is 200 mg of calcium per serving.

Examining the Critical Role of Vitamin D

You can't have healthy bones unless you take in enough vitamin D. Although you probably already know that calcium is essential to build strong bones, you may not realize that without vitamin D, your body can't properly absorb or utilize calcium (see Chapter 11 for more on vitamin D supplementation).

In many parts of the world, people easily obtain vitamin D through sunlight exposure, the main source of vitamin D. However, many elderly housebound people, as well as those cooped up in an office with nary a ray of sunlight exposure day after day, and those who live where it seems the sun rarely shines, may all be vitamin D deficient, unless they work at getting enough to compensate in their diet.

Fortunately, many processed foods are fortified with vitamin D. Companies began fortifying milk and cereals with vitamin D in the 1930s to help prevent *rickets,* a disease caused by vitamin D deficiency.

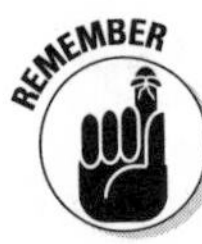

Milk is a good source of vitamin D only because manufacturers add vitamin D to the milk. Cows' milk alone has none! Because milk is a good source of vitamin D, you may assume that cheese and other dairy products, such as ice cream and yogurt, are also good sources, but only milk is artificially fortified with vitamin D. You won't find vitamin D in large quantities in other dairy products, so don't count your daily ice cream bar as a part of your vitamin D requirement! Vitamin D–fortified milk isn't used in the production of many other dairy products.

Because only certain foods are fortified with vitamin D, doctors are recognizing more and more patients with blood levels of vitamin D below the recommended amount. Years ago, doctors didn't have particularly accurate ways of measuring the amount of vitamin D in their patients' blood. Newer tests are more accurate.

To complicate matters, many foods have less vitamin D than they used to have. We believe (and there is literature to back this up) that vitamin D deficiency is becoming much more common among adults especially those living in northern climates. One cup of milk has about 100 International Units (IU) of vitamin D in it, but the minimum requirement is 200 IU daily. If you have osteoporosis, your doctor may recommend upwards of 800 IU of vitamin D daily.

So if you don't drink milk, if you're not exposed to enough sunlight, and if you don't take a multivitamin, you may be at risk for vitamin D deficiency. Other options do exist. For example, raisin bran is fortified with 77 IU of vitamin D, but the amount can vary from brand to brand. Table 5-7 lists some good food sources of vitamin D for you to consider.

Table 5-7 Important Food Sources of Vitamin D

Food *Add Milk*	*International Units (IU) Per Serving*
Cheese, 1 ounce	12 IU or less
Egg, 1 whole (yolk contains vitamin D)	20 IU
Fortified cereals, 1 serving	40 to 80 IU
Fortified margarine, 2 teaspoons	60 IU
Salmon, canned 3 ounces	360 IU
Liver, 3.5 ounces	30 IU

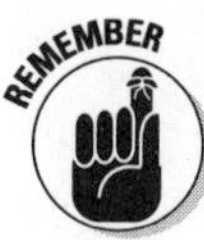

If you have reduced bone mineral density, have your doctor measure the vitamin D levels in your blood. Many experts consider a level less than 25 micrograms/dl to be abnormal. Years ago, experts in bone metabolism thought that this level might have been adequate, however new information suggests that more is better!

Nutrients You Probably Never Think About

The list of nutrients that affect your bones is staggering, so we just touch on a couple here.

- **Phosphorus:** Phosphorus in the form of phosphate makes up more than half of the mineral in bone, so you may think that phosphorus is good. It is — up to 700 mg a day. However, excess phosphorus, more than 3,000 to 4,000 mg daily, can result in calcium loss. A normal diet contains adequate phosphorus. You can find large amounts of phosphorus in soft drinks and many processed foods.

- **Potassium:** If you have a diet low in potassium, your body may overcompensate by removing calcium from your bones, thus weakening them. You can find potassium in fruits, vegetables, poultry, fish, milk, and yogurt.

Setting Down the Saltshaker

The United States is a nation of saltshaker addicts. Many (your coauthor Sharon shamefully included) often salt all their food without even tasting it first to see if the salt is even necessary.

Excess sodium chloride increases urinary calcium loss. If you're a saltshaker addict, your sodium intake is probably in the "excess" column! Several studies show that an additional gram of sodium a day increases calcium loss by 1 percent a year, unless you offset the loss with additional calcium intake.

Because high sodium intake is also associated with high blood pressure and water retention, you can do yourself a number of health-related favors simply by not using your saltshaker so enthusiastically. Keep your sodium intake down to 1 teaspoon of table salt daily, or 2,400 mg of sodium. If you have high blood pressure, kidney disease, or heart failure, discuss the amount of salt in your diet with your physician.

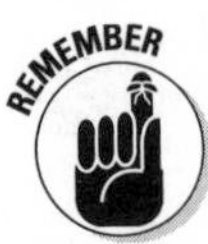

Don't forget to count the sodium found in processed foods. These amounts can be extremely high — as high as 420 mg in one can of "lowered-sodium" soup!

High Protein or Low Protein?

The debate over high protein diets as a good way to lose weight has enlarged to include questions on whether a high protein diet is good or bad for your bones.

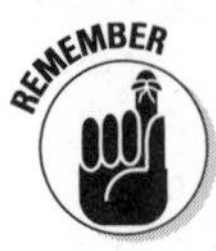

Protein is a necessary part of your diet. Men need 56 grams of protein a day, while women need 46 grams. Some studies have shown that taking in too little protein results in weak bones. And people who break their hip and who don't get enough protein are more likely to have a slow recovery with more medical problems.

But what about the opposite issue — taking in too high amounts of protein? If a little is good, is a lot better? Experts are debating this question. Several recent studies show that high protein diets can result in too much calcium being excreted in your urine, which can result in less calcium for your bones.

Looking at the acid test

The whole high protein versus osteoporosis issue revolves around acid, or more specifically, your body's acid-base balance.

Your body's *acidity* or *alkalinity* is expressed as pH, which stands for "potential of hydrogen." This level indicates the acidity or alkalinity of liquids. All liquids have a pH falling between 0 and 14. A pH of 7 is neutral, or balanced. A pH less than 7 is considered acidic; higher than 7 is considered alkaline.

Your body functions best when it's neither acidic nor alkaline — at a pH of 7, in other words. Different foods contain varying amounts of acid that may affect the acid-base balance in your body.

Recent studies show that a high intake of high acid nutrients, such as meat, can increase acidity in your body. To neutralize this acid, more minerals may need to be released from bone, resulting in weakened bone.

Researchers haven't done enough studies following people on high protein diets for a long period of time to conclude if they develop osteoporosis. Many factors can affect your excretion of calcium; some studies show that as long as your calcium intake is adequate, a high protein diet doesn't result in weakened bones.

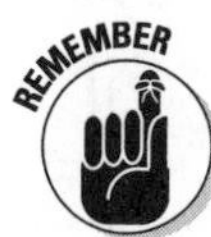

For now, the sensible approach to diet and osteoporosis is also the healthiest approach to diet in general: common sense and moderation. The best diet for overall health is one that emphasizes protein, vegetables, and fruit, and de-emphasizes sugar, processed foods, and soft drinks.

Assessing Alcohol in Your Diet

For many years, excess alcohol consumption has been known to be a risk factor for skeletal fractures especially among men. The question is how much alcohol is safe to drink, because some research has shown perhaps some beneficial effects of drinking small amounts of alcohol on cholesterol levels.

The problem is that 1 in 13 Americans abuse alcohol or are alcoholics. What happens to your bone in that situation? Drinking excess alcoholic beverages

- Disrupts your body's calcium balance
- Leaches calcium from bone

- Interferes with the conversion of vitamin D to its active form
- Lowers serum testosterone levels, which is a hormone important in bone strength in both men and women

Excess alcohol intake can also make you prone to falls. In one study of 84,000 women, moderate alcohol intake — more than one to two drinks per day — was associated with a higher risk of forearm and hip fractures.

Drinking too much alcohol can also lead to poor nutrition. Many alcoholics are deficient in nutrients due to poor diet.

So is drinking alcohol okay or not? If you're not normally a drinker, we probably don't see any reason to start now. But if you enjoy a glass of wine at night, restrict your intake to just one glass.

Decreasing Caffeine: Does it Matter?

Are you addicted to lattes? Do you need at least a pot of coffee to get you going each day? Can you not get by in the afternoons without a large, two-gallon jumbo cola? All are sources of caffeine, and although the buzz caffeine supplies may get you up and make you feisty, it may also leach calcium from your bones.

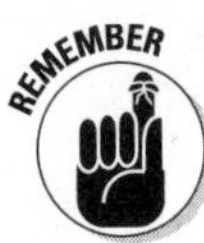

Excess caffeine intake may disturb your body's balance of calcium and phosphorus, which can cause increased calcium loss in your urine. The phosphoric acid found in many soft drinks has the same effect, resulting in a loss of calcium for your bones. Coffee and soft drinks aren't the only culprits. Don't forget that some over-the-counter medication, such as Excedrin, contains significant amounts of caffeine.

Studies show that a moderate intake of caffeine, up to four cups of coffee a day, doesn't increase bone loss. This doesn't mean you can have four of the double lattes, each served in a cup the size of Texas, and think you're within your daily caffeine allowance! A cup is 8 ounces of regular coffee. If you consume more than that (include cola intake), you need to consider cutting back. One way to offset calcium excretion due to caffeine intake is to put a little calcium-containing dairy product into each cup of coffee. We can't recommend this for cola addicts, however!

If you're a caffeine junkie, you need extra calcium to replace the excess amounts being excreted in your urine. (See Chapter 11 about taking calcium supplements.)

Looking At How Your Weight Affects Your Bones

Thick or thin, fat or skinny, what's best for your bones? Because most other health issues say thin is better, you may assume the same is true for your bones, but that's not necessarily the case. Excessive dieting isn't good when it comes to osteoporosis.

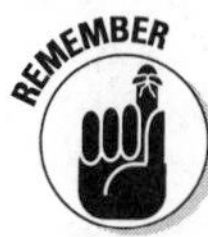

Some studies show that thin women who are overly concerned about their weight and diet frequently have bone density that is 6 percent lower than women of average weight. If your weight drops below 127 pounds, your physician needs to be appropriately concerned that you're at higher risk for development of osteoporosis.

Clearly, obsessive dieting to the point of anorexia or *amenorrhea* (lack of menstrual periods, caused by low estrogen levels) can result in low bone density that may last a lifetime. (See Chapter 4 for more on anorexia.) Plenty of low calorie sources of calcium are available to keep you both trim and bone-strong at the same time.

What about the other side of the coin, that is, being overweight? "Fat" has a negative connotation in the United States and elsewhere. And even though "fat" in the sense of true obesity is certainly bad for your health, some fat is necessary. Research has shown that higher body weight can influence bone mass through four mechanisms:

- Larger mechanical loading
- More muscle mass
- Higher levels of sex hormones
- Less bone resorption

Estrogen levels in your body are related to fat, and estrogen helps build strong bones by decreasing bone breakdown and helping maintain adequate levels of vitamin D.

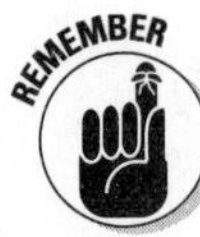

Osteoporosis is actually less common in overweight people, but that's hardly a reason to gain large amounts of weight, because the risks of obesity on many other body functions are well documented. The bottom line for adults is that you need to discuss your proper weight with your physician. Too much is harmful. Too little is harmful as well.

With regard to children, weight issues may be different. Some recent studies have shown that overweight children have lower bone density than their normal weight peers. Their lower exercise levels and decreased intake of calcium and increased amounts of carbonated beverages may account for these findings.

You can help your overweight child develop better bone density by cutting out sodas and substituting low-fat milk. Encourage your child to be active; your child may never make the Olympics, and may not want to play competitive sports, but cycling, weight lifting, or just walking can pay big dividends in stronger bones. Better yet, go out with your child when he exercises, and you'll develop not only stronger bones, but also a closer relationship with your kid.

Chapter 6

Exercising for Strong Bones

In This Chapter

- Taking the first steps to exercise
- Exercising and loving it
- Determining how to fit exercise into your life
- Steering clear of injuries
- Following through with your exercise plan

Having a love-hate relationship with the idea of exercise is so easy. You may fully realize the obvious health benefits of a regular exercise program, yet dread the idea of devoting time to what you're sure is a mundane activity.

We can promise, however, that as soon as you start and actually carry out an exercise routine, the health and psychological benefits will be so obvious that you'll greatly miss your exercise routine when you can't perform it. In other words — try it, you'll probably like it!

Experts agree that weight-bearing exercise benefits your bones. You may worry that exercising when you have osteoporosis is dangerous, or that exercise might cause more fractures, but the opposite is actually true. The right exercises actually strengthen your bones and decrease your chance of fracture.

In this chapter, we discuss what exercises are best to prevent or lessen osteoporosis, how to set up and actually continue an exercise plan, how to avoid injuries after you're on the plan, and how to keep a smile on your face while doing something that's great for your bones!

Starting While You're Still Young

When's the best time to start an exercise program to prevent osteoporosis? Yesterday! Actually, the best time to start is at birth; building bone is a lifelong proposition.

Most of you remember childhood as a time of physical activity — roller-skating, jumping rope, riding bikes, climbing hills, and swimming were a daily part of life. Sadly, as people age they become less active. In fact, studies show that by age 16, only a little more than 10 percent of girls are involved in regular physical activity. As a matter of fact, the Surgeon General's report in 2002 stated that only 25 percent of U.S. high-school students participated in daily physical education, down from 42 percent in the early 1990s.

Although you may want to blame video games and TV for the decrease in physical activity in young children as well as teens, parents (and grandparents) need to take some responsibility. Parents are the ones who control the on-off switch on electronic equipment. If you're a parent (or grandparent), pull the plug and encourage your kids (and grandkids) to go outside and play instead of spending all their time killing intergalactic invaders. Children and teens need to be involved in one hour each day of moderate to vigorous activity, and moving the computer mouse doesn't qualify!

Better yet — get up off the couch and join them in biking, hiking, or inline skating. (Make sure you check with your doctor before starting any exercise program, and make sure your health insurance is current if you haven't exercised in a while!)

Even though you may think it's too late for you to relive your childhood and keep physical activity on your daily calendar, it's not too late to influence the next generation — your children and grandchildren. Active children tend to have active parents — and grandparents, too! Stay active with your kids and grandkids by taking hikes, riding bikes, dancing, or swimming. You can reap some benefits for yourself and also help them avoid any future problems with osteoporosis.

Even if you're starting to gray, you need regular exercise. Exercise is not only good for osteoporosis, but it also helps your heart, your lungs, your mental outlook, your sex life (va-va-va-voom!), and the way your clothes fit!

Moving Your Bones to Build More Bone

Does it sound odd that using your bones actually makes them stronger? Doesn't it at least seem logical that using your bones wears them out faster? That's not the case though.

Why do you need to use exercise to build bone instead of just relying on medication? Three reasons come to mind. Exercise is

- Inexpensive
- Effective
- Good for you and provides additional health benefits

Understanding why exercise strengthens bone

Exercise that moves your muscles stimulates your bones. As the muscle pulls against the bone it's attached to, it stimulates the bone to rebuild and become dense. One reason for this is that your bone, like every other part of you, adapts to a certain level of activity. When you increase that activity level, you increase blood flow to your bones, which results in increased nutrients for growth going to your bones.

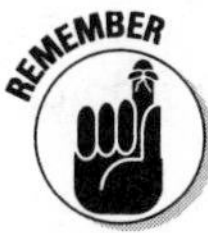

Building muscle helps build bone. Although exercise won't completely prevent you from losing bone, it can help slow the process. In addition, exercise can

- Strengthen muscles and reduce pain
- Improve your sense of balance and decrease your chance of falling
- Better your overall health

Utilizing weight-bearing exercise and resistance training

Weight-bearing exercise and resistance training are both beneficial for increasing muscle and bone mass and avoiding fractures.

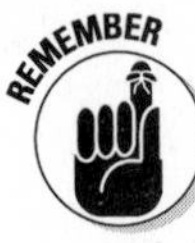

Weight bearing refers to any exercise that places your full weight on your legs. In other words, if you're standing, you're weight bearing! However, if you're just standing there, you're not exercising. Weight-bearing exercise means using your bones and muscles to work against gravity when you move.

Gravity keeps you on earth instead of letting you float through the air like an astronaut. Because gravity is holding you down, it takes effort to move your muscles and bones against it. If you're moving against gravity while standing up, you're doing weight-bearing exercise. Some examples of weight-bearing exercise are running, walking, stair climbing, dancing, jumping rope, jogging in place, or playing sports, such as tennis, volleyball, or racquetball.

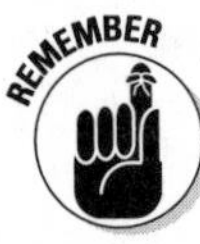

Meanwhile, resistance training includes any activity that involves overcoming resistance, such as pushing, pulling, or lifting. Some examples of resistance training are lifting weights, doing push-ups or pull-ups, or using specially designed exercise machines that allow you to push or pull against a set resistance level.

Resistance exercise helps bone grow because the tendon the bone is attached to pulls on the bone, encouraging bone-cell activity. As your muscles become stronger, they continue to stress the bones, stimulating more bone-building cells to grow.

Because water doesn't create much resistance or allow weight bearing, swimming isn't classified in either of these categories. However, because water exercise is good for your heart and muscle strength, it's a good choice of exercise for many people, especially those unable to bear weight on joints because of pain or other problems.

Developing an Exercise Plan

Okay, you've decided to start exercising. You've bought a bike, a jump rope, three jogging suits, and a pair of inline skates, and you've signed up for 90 sessions a month at the gym. Are you ready? No, you're not! Take off those skates! You need to spend some time planning a serious exercise program before you go flying off in a dozen directions, some of which may well result in muscle strain, if not a few broken bones!

Remember that the key to an exercise program, or any other program, is a reality check. What can you realistically do? What *should* you realistically do? Although it seems obvious, most people skip an important first step — talking to their doctor.

Having healthy bones isn't going to do you any good if you exercise yourself into collapse during the first week! Before you start buying out the sporting goods store, ask yourself and your doctor a few questions, such as:

- **Do I have any physical limitations on exercise?** If you've lived a few years, you probably have some wounded areas. How about the hand you broke three times playing racquetball, the knee you twisted playing football, and the foot you had surgery on last year? Most of you have a "weak spot" acquired from years of daily living. Try not to aggravate any existing problems when you start exercising.
- **Is there any kind of exercise I shouldn't be doing?** The restrictions may be health related. For example, if you have exercise-induced asthma, running probably isn't a good activity. If you have heart problems, your doctor may not want you undertaking certain types of exercise.

  Restrictions can also be common-sense restrictions. For example, if you live on a major highway, jogging may not be a good choice, unless you can go to a track somewhere. Ice-skating is impractical if you live in Hawaii, unless you have an indoor rink nearby.
- **What do I enjoy doing?** Suffice it to say that if you like what you're doing, you'll probably keep doing it, and if you hate what you're doing, you'll probably stop at the first muscle twinge.
- **How much will it cost?** Unfortunately, cost is a major factor in many people's exercise plan. Gym memberships and sports equipment can be expensive. Even walking can add up if, like your co-author Sharon, you require expensive specialized athletic shoes!

Setting an exercise schedule

If you try to do too much too fast, you may end up wearing yourself out or even hurting yourself. If you overdo it at the beginning, you may end up not doing any exercise at all in the long run.

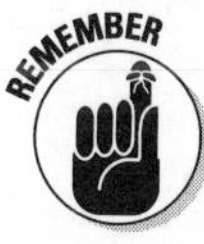

Setting a schedule for exercise requires that you look *realistically* at your schedule. If you plan to spend every lunch hour at the gym from now until Christmas, don't forget to factor in your once-a-week lunch hour with your friends from high school and the garden club's weekly meeting. Are you really going to avoid all lunchtime social engagements for the rest of your life, or even for a month?

If you're like most people, the answer is no. So be realistic. If you can plan to spend three days a week at the gym, with some time on the treadmill at home another day or two, you'll still be way ahead.

Don't feel like you need to do all your exercise at one time, either. A walk at lunch and a bike ride with your kids after work adds up to an hour a day, but it doesn't feel like you're spending all your time exercising. Get creative — just make sure you get active!

Finding time in your life for exercise

If you're working and your lunch hours are nonexistent, then you need to squeeze exercise into some other time of the day. Many gyms open early so that you can exercise before work. Going in the morning may be a better plan than going after work, when all you want to do is go home and collapse, *if* you're motivated enough to get up in the morning to go to the gym and make it to work on time.

If you're a caretaker at home, finding time to get to the gym may be difficult. Even though many gyms have childcare on-site, few have eldercare. Being the caregiver for a parent or a disabled spouse can affect your exercise schedule, and you may need to keep your exercise regimen close to home.

One way to keep your family active and also spend quality time together is to make exercise a family affair. How about bikes for the whole bunch — and a baby carrier on the back for your youngest member? Or just take a walk with your little guys — pushing the stroller provides great resistance training!

Avoiding Injury While Exercising

You may be prone to initial hyperenthusiasm about exercising. Or are you the type of person who has to be dragged, kicking and screaming, into the gym? For people who begin any new project with incredible amounts of misdirected enthusiasm, we need to insert a word of warning here.

Overdoing exercise when you're not used to it can cause muscle damage that can permanently sideline you from the Macarena line. Start slowly and work up to a more strenuous routine, and utilize the gym's trainers to help you pick the machines that will benefit you most. Of course, the trainer can also coach you to use the machines correctly. You can damage your muscles by exercising

Don't let the muscleheads intimidate you

Does the thought of walking into the gym alone scare you to death? Find a friend or drag your partner with you so you can discover how to exercise correctly together (people typically don't feel as foolish when they have an equally inept partner with them) and also can cheer each other on.

Even if you go in a group of ten, you may find the gym intimidating at first. Some gyms now cater just to women, or to the over-40 crowd, so don't feel like the local Beefy Studs R Us Gym Inc. is your only option. Visit a few places to get a feel for the clientele before signing on any dotted lines.

Don't be scared off, though, if everyone you see is fit and trim. After all, that's what you want to be too! Invest in a workout outfit or two if you feel conspicuous in the sweats you've owned since high school. Make sure you're comfortable in everything so you don't have to worry about parts of your outfit riding up or down during your workout.

incorrectly, not to mention the damage you'll do if you drop weights on your foot by mistake! Find out how to do exercises properly from the beginning; your bones, muscles, and tendons will all thank you!

Getting Down to the Nitty-Gritty: Choosing an Exercise Routine

Sooner or later, you need to get down to business. All the running shoes and color-coordinated outfits won't help a bit until you start putting them to use. To get started, pick a time, starting with 20 to 30 minutes a day, three days a week, as a recommendation. Then pick an activity from the following list, and end your routine with 15 minutes of weight training, also known as strength or resistance training.

Some weight-bearing cardiovascular workouts include

- Cross-country skiing
- Dancing
- Jumping rope
- Light jogging (make sure your knees are up to this!)

- Playing tennis
- Stair climbing
- Walking outside or on a treadmill

Do you want to painlessly increase your daily cardiovascular workout? Take the stairs instead of the elevator every chance you get — and park at the back of the parking lot, instead of circling around looking for the spot closest to the door.

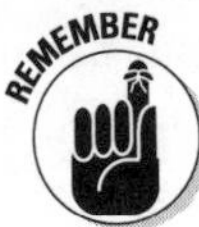

Weight, or resistance, training allows you to be specific about the bones you want to strengthen, so you want to add exercises targeting your hips, spine, and arms — the most frequent fracture sights in osteoporosis. Weight training may give you a mental picture of rippling muscles lifting a hundred pounds over their owner's head, but weight training can be very simple; you don't even need to buy weights. You can use anything that's easy to hold, as long as you have two of them so you work both arms equally.

Resistance training has benefits beyond bone building. A study done at the University of Florida's Colleges of Medicine and Health and Human Performance showed that people working with weights three times a week for six months were able to work out longer on a treadmill.

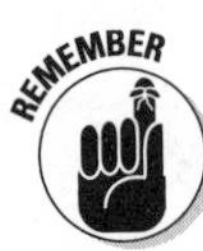

When you begin resistance training, start with one- to two-pound weights and work up gradually. If you can't comfortably do eight repetitions of an exercise, the weight you're using is too heavy. If you can do more than 15 repetitions easily, it's too light. For some of you, you may not be able to use any weights at all to start! Build up at your own pace.

Follow these easy steps when using weights:

1. **Take three seconds to lift the weights, and then hold in position for one second.**
2. **Lower over another three seconds.**
3. **Breathe slowly, exhaling as you lift and inhaling as you lower the weight.**
4. **Do one set of 8 to 15 repetitions (reps), starting with 8 to 12 reps and working up to 12 to 15 reps.**
5. **Rest for 30 to 60 seconds, and then do a second set.**

Don't forget to start with a weight you can lift only eight times. Stay at that weight until you can lift it 12 to 15 times. Then add weight until, once again, you can lift it only eight times. Add more weight each time you can easily do 12 to 15 reps.

Don't exercise the same group of muscles two days in a row — alternate exercises to allow muscles to recover.

Biceps curls with dumbbells

Biceps curls work your upper outer arms, or *biceps.* Biceps work to bend your arm. Start cautiously if you have lower back or elbow problems.

Doing the exercise

1. **Hold a dumbbell in each hand and stand with your feet as far apart as the width of your hips.**

   You can also do this exercise sitting in a chair.

2. **Keep your arms at your sides with palms facing your body.**

   (See Figure 6-1.)

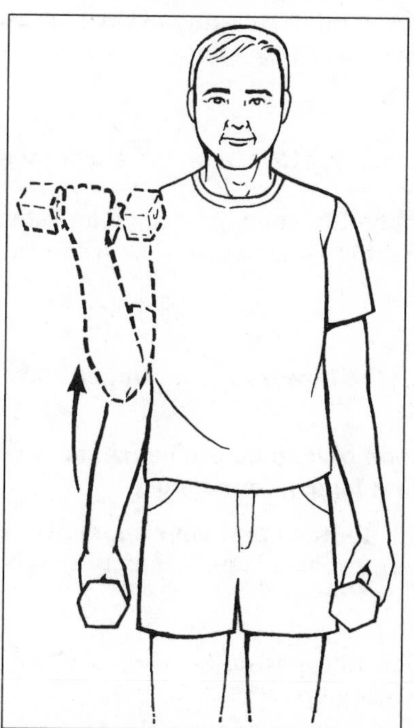

Figure 6-1: Keep your elbows close to your body for the entire exercise.

3. **Bend your right arm up, keeping it close to your shoulder.**

   Turn your palm as you lift so that it's facing your shoulder at the top of the movement.

4. **Lower the dumbbell slowly; repeat with your left hand.**

   (See Figure 6-1.)

Doing it correctly

Do:

- Keep your elbows close to your body.
- Keep your knees relaxed and back straight.
- Lower the weight slowly; don't just let it fall back.

Triceps kickback

Triceps kickback works your *triceps,* which are the upper inner part of your arm. Triceps work to straighten your arm. Start slowly if you have elbow or lower back problems.

Doing the exercise

You need a bench or something to lean on to do this exercise.

1. **Hold your dumbbell in your right hand and stand with your left side next to your bench — or whatever you're using to lean on.**

   (See Figure 6-2.)

2. **Lean forward at the hips until your upper body is at a 45-degree angle.**
3. **Use your left hand to lean on the bench, or whatever you're using for a bench, for support.**
4. **Bend your right elbow so that your upper arm is parallel to the floor, your forearm is perpendicular to it, and your palm faces in.**

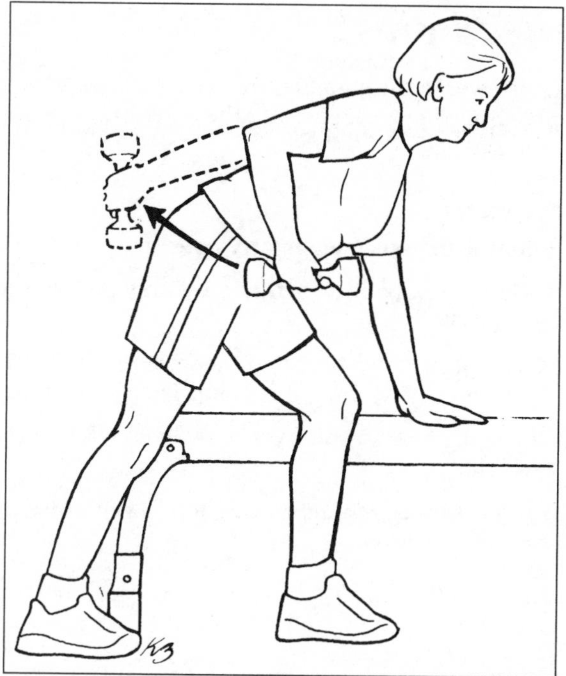

Figure 6-2: Don't let your upper arm move or your shoulder drop below waist level.

5. **Hold your upper arm still and straighten your arm until the end of your dumbbell is pointing straight down.**
6. **Slowly bend your arm to lower the weight.**
7. **Repeat with your left arm after you complete the set.**

   (Refer to Figure 6-2.)

Doing it correctly

Do:

- Keep your abdominal muscles pulled in and your knees relaxed.
- Straighten your arm but keep your elbow relaxed.
- Hold your upper arm still.
- Keep your shoulder above waist level.

Overhead press

This exercise works the shoulder muscles (*deltoids*), the upper back (*upper trapezius*), triceps, and the sides of rib cage (the *oblique* muscles).

Doing the exercise

1. **Stand with your feet slightly apart.**
2. **Hold a dumbbell in each hand with your arms at shoulder height.**

   Keep your elbows bent and the weights about six inches from your body, with your palms facing outward.
3. **Slowly lift the weight over your head with your arm straight.**
4. **Hold for three seconds, and then lower slowly to your starting position.**

   (Check out Figure 6-3.)

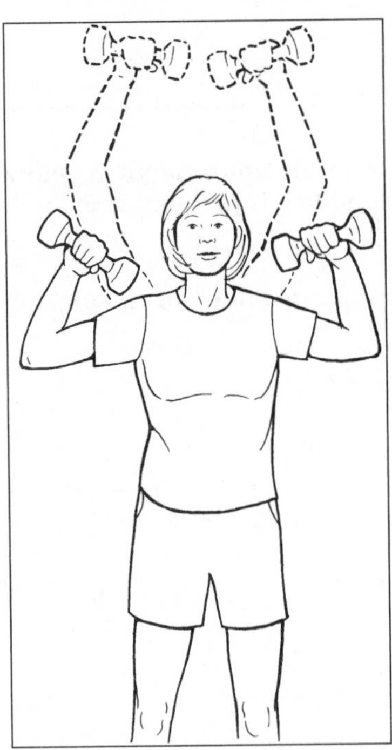

Figure 6-3: Be sure to hold the weights so your palms are facing outwards.

Doing it correctly

Do:

- Keep your back straight.
- Keep your knees relaxed.
- Hold for less than three seconds if you're afraid you're going to drop the weights on your head!

Knee extensors

Knee extensors work your hips and legs to help strengthen them. Never bounce your leg while doing this exercise, or you'll tighten the muscles unnecessarily and risk a knee injury.

As your legs get stronger through your exercise routines, you may want to purchase some ankle weights to help continue increasing your strength. Ankle weights are soft weights, about ten pounds each, that strap around your ankles with Velcro. You can usually find them in any store that carries athletic equipment.

Doing the exercise

You need a chair or something to sit on to do this exercise.

1. **Sit in the chair with your knees six inches apart and a small, rolled hand towel under your lower thigh to elevate it *slightly*.**
2. **Slowly lift your right foot until your leg is straight out in front of you, and then slowly lower your foot back down to the floor.**
3. **Repeat 8 to 15 times for each leg.**

   (See Figure 6-4.)

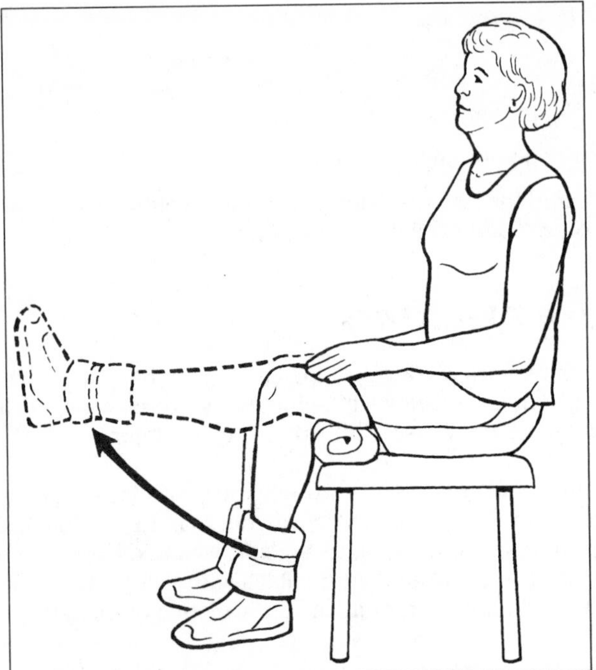

Figure 6-4: The proper way to do knee extensors.

Doing it correctly

Do:

- Keep your abdominal muscles pulled in.
- Lift from the knee, not from the hip.
- Move slowly and make sure not to jerk your knees.

Hip extensors

This exercise goes a long way toward strengthening your hips and legs.

Doing the exercise

You need a sturdy chair to lean on for balance. You also need the ankle weights that we mention in the "Knee extensors" exercise in the previous section.

1. **Holding onto the back of the chair, bend forward at your waist at about a 45-degree angle.**

2. **Slowly lift one leg behind you as straight as you can and as high as possible.**
3. **Slowly lower your leg back down to the floor.**
4. **Repeat 8 to 15 times with each leg.**

   (Check out Figure 6-5.)

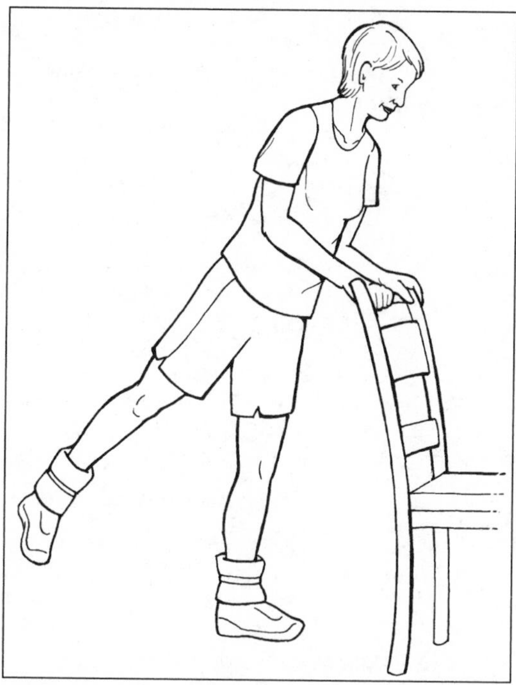

Figure 6-5: The proper way to do hip extensors.

Doing it correctly

Do:

- Keep your legs straight.
- Make sure to not bend your upper body when lifting your leg.
- Build up your repetitions as you get stronger.

Hip flexors

Hip flexors help strengthen your hips and legs.

Doing the exercise

You need a sturdy chair to hold onto for balance. You can also use ankle weights as you progress.

1. **Holding onto the back of the chair, slowly bring your knee as close to your chest as you can without bending your other knee or your waist.**

   (See Figure 6-6.)

2. **Slowly lower your leg back to the floor, repeating 8 to 15 times on each side.**

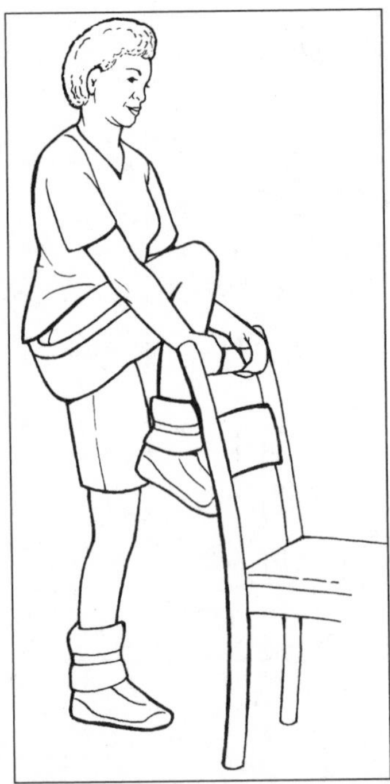

Figure 6-6: The proper way to do hip flexors.

Doing it correctly

Do:

- Keep the knee you're not lifting straight.
- Keep your back straight.
- Lower your leg slowly.
- Add ankle weights as you build up strength.

Leg lifts

Leg lifts help build your leg, abdominal, and hip muscles.

Doing the exercise

You need a chair to sit on. Add ankle weights as you build strength,

1. **Sit on a chair and slide forward until your buttocks are near the edge of the seat.**

   Support yourself by holding on to the seat with both hands.

2. **Lift both feet together two to three inches off the floor and hold for two seconds.**

   (See Figure 6-7.)

3. **Slowly lower legs to the floor.**

   Repeat 8 to 15 times.

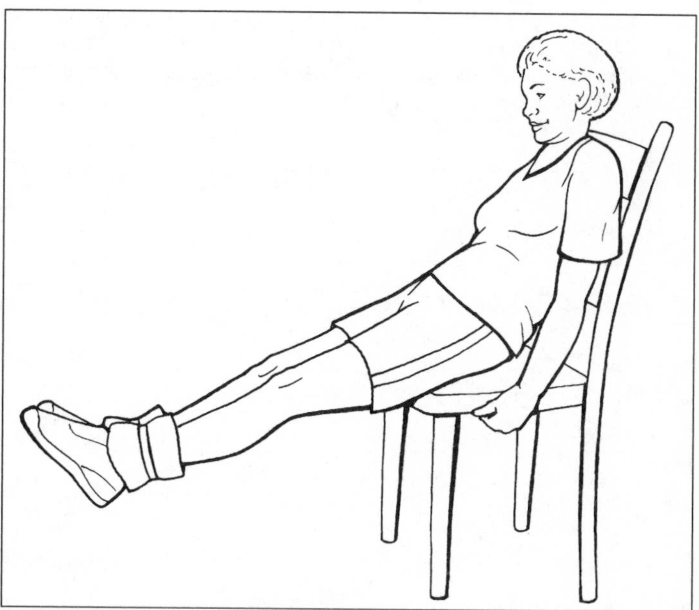

Figure 6-7: The proper way to do leg lifts.

Doing it correctly

Do:

- Hold on to the sides of the chair so you don't slide to the floor!
- Add ankle weights as you build up strength.
- Raise your legs a little higher as you build strength.

If you've experienced spinal compression fractures, avoid any exercises that flex the spine. If you suffer from these types of fractures, start exercising under a physical therapist's guidance. (See Chapters 7 and 13 for more info on spinal compression fractures.)

If you're interested in more information about exercising, you can check out *Weight Training For Dummies,* 2nd Edition, by Liz Neporent and Suzanne Schlosberg, or *Cross-Training For Dummies* by Tony Ryan and Martica Heaner (both by Wiley).

You can also check out an excellent videotape by the National Institute on Aging available at `http://www.niapublications.org/exercisevideo/index.asp`. The 48-minute video, called *Exercise: A Video from the National Institute on Aging,* also comes with a companion booklet.

Part III
Diagnosing and Treating Osteoporosis

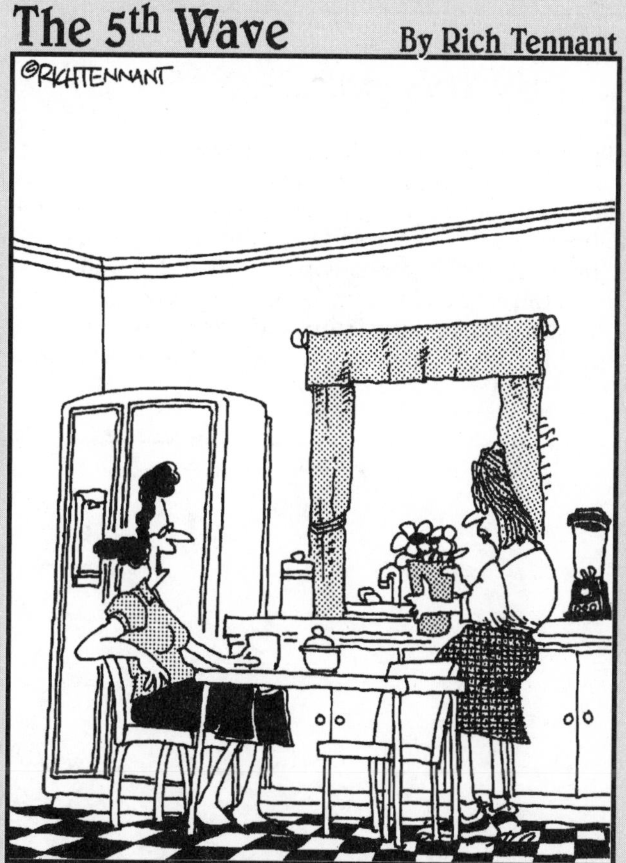

"Right now I'm exercising pain management through medication, meditation, and limiting visits from my pain-in-the-butt neighbor."

In this part . . .

If you're worried about having osteoporosis and don't know where to go for help or what to expect in the way of treatment, you're in the right place! In this part, we tell you how to find a doctor and what the latest treatments and medications are for osteoporosis. We also walk you through the care and treatment of broken bones. Finally, we sneak a peek into the future and preview the new treatments and diagnostic tools that may eliminate osteoporosis in the next generation.

Chapter 7

Facing the Consequences of Bones Gone Bad

In This Chapter

- Realizing that bone loss is a silent disease
- Understanding fragility fractures
- Name that fracture: Knowing which bone is broken

You're probably quite aware that aging brings changes to your fragile skin; the proof is in the mirror every day. Although you don't visibly see the changes to your insides like you see the wrinkles on the outside, those internal changes are there nonetheless.

Similar to many of the other changes that come with increasing age, people don't notice the changes in their bones until it's too late. In other words, osteoporosis is a silent disease. You don't have any pain until you break a bone!

In this chapter, we explain the different types of fractures that you can experience when you have osteoporosis and the types of problems that can occur as a result. Knowing how and why bones break in osteoporosis is the first step in understanding how to prevent fractures.

Aging and Your Bones

As we discuss in Chapter 2, bones are beautifully engineered and marvelously efficient — until something goes awry. You first need to understand why keeping your bones strong and healthy is so important.

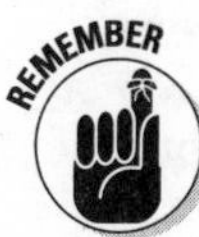

Early detection and preventive treatment before fractures occur is the vital key to treating osteoporosis. (Check out Chapter 3 for the best ways to keep your bones strong.)

Osteoporosis is somewhat similar to high blood pressure (hypertension). For instance, if you have high blood pressure, you may not know it, because people rarely experience any symptoms from an elevated blood pressure. Untreated hypertension causes damage to blood vessels over many years. But if high blood pressure is diagnosed early, its devastating consequences (stroke and heart disease) can be prevented.

When you develop a fracture from osteoporosis, it's likely that you have had the problem for years. In other words, by the time you have an osteoporotic fracture, bone is already quite fragile. You can lose bone at the rate of 5 percent per year (for example during menopause) and not experience any pain at all. So unless you discover you have osteoporosis at an early stage, before you have any symptoms (see Chapter 9), you'll already have weak bones at the time of your first symptom, which can be a devastating and even life-threatening fracture.

Don't get the impression that as soon as a fracture occurs, no treatment can help. Studies have shown that bone density can improve even at later stages, and fracture rates can be reduced. A recent estimate by the Office of the Surgeon General reports that by the year 2020, nearly one-half of Americans will be at risk for developing fractures, if doctors don't make changes in their approach to early diagnosis and treatment of osteoporosis. Table 7-1 shows what the lifetime risk of fracture is broken down by age and gender.

Table 7-1 Lifetime Risk of Fracture at Age 50: Men and Women

Type of Fracture	*Men*	*Women*
Arm	2.5 percent	16 percent
Hip	6 percent	17.5 percent
Spine	5 percent	15.6 percent

Facing Fragility Fractures

Your doctor may often use the phrase "fragility fracture" when you experience a broken bone with minimal trauma. You probably know that experiencing a fracture with normal, healthy, strong bones is certainly possible. For instance, a child who falls from a tree and fractures an arm can have normal bone strength, but the impact is still too great to withstand a break. On the other hand, people with osteoporosis or other problems, such as *osteomalacia* (adult rickets), can develop a fracture without a significant injury.

Hip fractures, vertebral compression fractures, and wrist fractures all should alert your physician to investigate your situation carefully and further delve into the possibility of you having lost bone strength. In infancy, the occurrence of multiple fractures should alert your pediatrician to the possibility of osteogenesis imperfecta. (See Chapter 4 for more on osteogenesis imperfecta.)

Your doctor also may diagnosis osteoporosis if you're unfortunate enough to require surgery on a broken bone. During surgery, your orthopedic surgeon can directly assess your bone quality. She may call a consultation after the procedure because your bones appear thin during the operation "like potato chips." You don't want to hear this term when describing your bones, do you? (And to think, you don't get any sour cream and chive dip to go with them.)

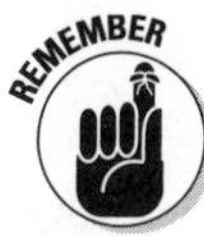

Increasing evidence suggests that any fracture in women *or* men older than 55 can be the first indication of a metabolic bone problem. Other fractures seen in osteoporosis include rib fractures, fractures of the arm (*humerus*), and pelvic bone fractures.

Finally, multiple fractures, even *with* significant trauma, should alert your physician to the *possibility* of a metabolic bone disease and prompt referral to a specialist.

For example, one of your co-author's nephews experienced three fractures over a two-year period while playing ice hockey. His doctors started him on vitamin D supplements, because he lived in New Hampshire, where the exposure to sunlight is variable. He hasn't had a fracture since!

Breaking Bones – Different Types of Fractures

Certain types of fractures are more commonly associated with osteoporosis and other bone diseases. In this section we define these common fracture types and the difficulties they can cause.

Falling on outstretched arms

Wrist fractures, often called *Colles' fractures,* typically occur as a result of osteoporosis. These breaks usually happen in the radius, the ulna, or some of the other small bones in your wrist (see Figure 7-1). Colles' fractures often occur when you fall and put your arm out to break your fall.

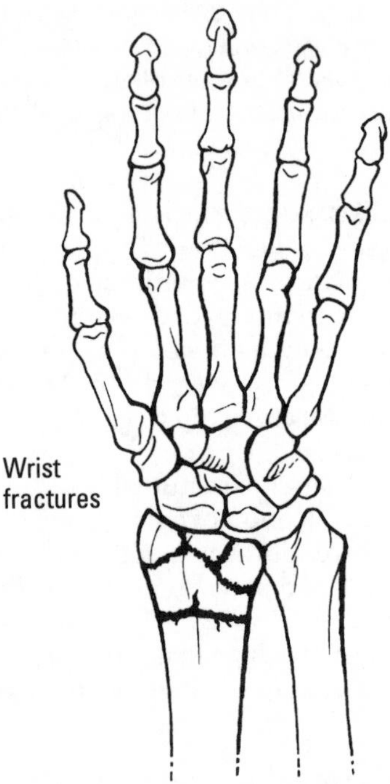

Figure 7-1: A wrist or Colles' fracture is very common in people with osteoporosis. Darker lines show where the wrist might break.

Treatment requires casting or some other form of immobilization. Sometimes you may require surgery. You may experience loss of motion of your wrist, but this type of fracture isn't nearly as devastating as a hip or spinal fracture.

However, the occurrence of a wrist fracture is clearly a warning sign that you may have an overall reduction in the strength of your bones. A Colles' fracture is therefore considered a *fragility fracture,* and your doctor needs to evaluate you for the possibility of osteoporosis or other bone disorders.

Who are more prone to wrist fractures? Among American women, the incidence of wrist fractures increases rapidly at the time of menopause and plateaus at about 700 per 100,000 persons per year after age 60.

"I broke my hip! Or was it my femur?"

What is commonly referred to as a "broken hip" is actually a fracture of the *femur,* the longest and heaviest bone in your body. The fracture is usually found at the neck of the femur, where it connects to the pelvis.

More than 300,000 people fracture their hip each year in the United States. In fact, hip fractures (see Figure 7-2) are the second most common type of osteoporotic fracture.

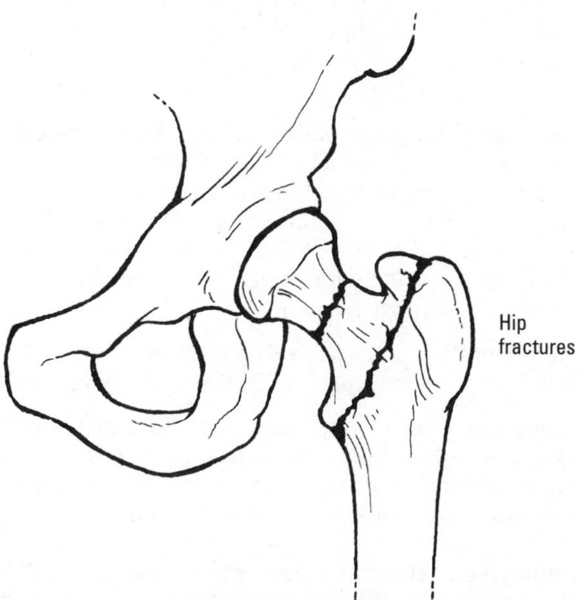

Figure 7-2: A "hip fracture" is actually a fracture of the femur, oftentimes in the *femoral neck,* which is an area that is particularly weak.

Ninety percent of all hip fractures are related to osteoporosis. Hip fractures are devastating and can have long-term consequences. A hip fracture

- **Requires a trip to the emergency room.** In the United States, in 1995, hip fractures resulted in 800,000 visits to emergency rooms.
- **Requires hospitalization with period of immobility.** In 2003, in the United States, there were 300,000 hospital admissions for hip fracture (defined as a fracture of the head of the

femur) in one year. There could be more fractures not included in this analysis.

- **Often requires surgery.** You need a new hip or a pin in your hip. (See Chapter 13 for more details about the surgery after hip fractures.) Surgery on your hip can be complicated by very serious problems including infection, pneumonia, and blood clots in your legs or lungs.

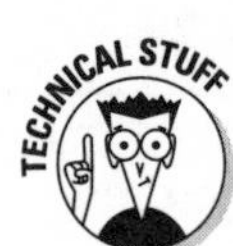

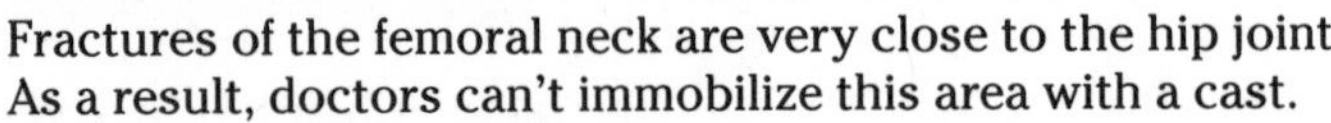

Fractures of the femoral neck are very close to the hip joint. As a result, doctors can't immobilize this area with a cast.

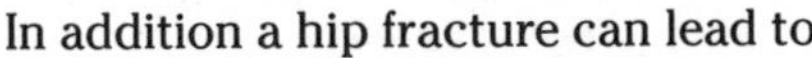

In addition a hip fracture can lead to

- **Increased disability from hip surgery.** One-fourth of all people with a hip fracture become disabled in the year after their fracture. Hip fractures result yearly in more than 7 million days of reduced activity.
- **Increased chance of ending up in a long-term care facility.** Almost 75 percent of all nursing home admissions are related to hip fractures from osteoporosis, which accounts for approximately 6,000 admissions yearly. Almost half the expense of hip fracture healthcare is paid to nursing homes. (In 1995, 180,000 people ended up in a chronic care facility because of a hip fracture.)
- **Reduced life expectation.** Hip fracture affects your health and ability to care for yourself (your risk of dying even!).

  If you were able to get around without a walker or other aid at the time of your hip fracture, fracturing you hip will almost triple (2.8 times) your risk of dying in the next three months, compared to people who don't have a fracture.

According to one study of women older than 65, each standard deviation decrease in bone density at the hip resulted in a 30 percent increase in total mortality. (See Chapter 9 for more info on standard deviations and bone density testing.)

Although we aren't intending to scare you, we want you to be aware that hip fractures are serious health problems that can result in your dying sooner than you would have without a fracture. The key is to avoid fracturing a hip. How can you stay alive longer by being fracture free? Prevention, prevention, prevention!

Falling and hip fractures

"Grandma fell and broke her hip." You've undoubtedly heard someone say this or you've even said it yourself. She actually fractured her femur, probably near the femoral neck.

Some studies show that occasionally people don't "fall and break their bone" at all. Instead they have a fracture of the femur from the simple stress of putting their foot down on a step. So the fracture causes the fall and not the other way around! How often this actually happens is difficult to say. Nonetheless, people in the healthcare field definitely want to prevent as many falls as possible by changing the environment and preventing hazards.

Some people are more prone to falling than others; they have what's known as *postural instability.* Your co-author Sharon is one of these people. If you're one, you undoubtedly already know it. You may walk into walls and trip over a crack in the sidewalk. Doctors aren't quite sure what causes postural instability, but it may be because you have visual issues, don't judge spatial relationships well, can't decipher depth perception, or have poor contrast sensitivity.

Whatever your reason for being spatially challenged (or as your grandchild may say, a klutz), you need to be especially careful when you have osteoporosis. If you're a klutz, you *know* you're going to fall or trip sooner or later, and every fall increases your chance for injury.

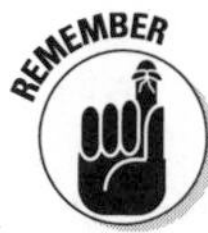

The Centers for Disease Control (CDC) statistics indicate that one-third of all people older than 65 fall each year, and that the majority of fractures result from falls. The good news is that most falls occur in your own home.

Why is this good news? It's good news, because you can control your own environment. You can't control the supermarket that mops aisle one and forgets to put out a "Be Careful" sign, but you can determine where you place your furniture and the kind of rugs you have on your stairs. (See Chapter 13 for more on falling and fractures.) You can also take preventive measures to avoid a fall. (And make sure to stay off that ladder!)

What's a stress fracture?

Many older people who fall can't really explain how they got to the ground. A spontaneous break in the femoral neck that results in a fall is called a stress fracture. We really don't know how many hip fractures are due to stress fractures and how many are due to an impact to the bone from hitting the ground.

Developing a dowager's hump

The phrase "dowager's hump" paints a vivid picture. You may think of your great-aunt or great-grandmother instantly, because you imagine an elderly woman with loss of height, hunched forward with a forward curvature of the spine. A *dowager's hump* is caused by compression fractures of the spine, called vertebral compression fractures.

A *compression fracture* is a break of the vertebrae in your back that typically changes the height of the vertebral body. Multiple compression fractures (see Figure 7-3) can result in a loss of up to five inches in height.

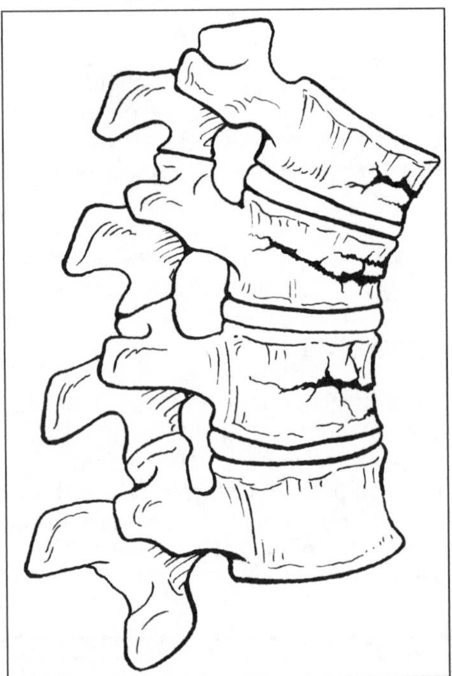

Figure 7-3: Compression fractures are responsible for the loss of height in many people with osteoporosis.

The dowager's hump appearance, more technically known as *kyphosis,* is caused by the inner part of the vertebrae collapsing. This creates what is known as a wedge fracture (see Figure 7-4) and can result in the spine bending forward.

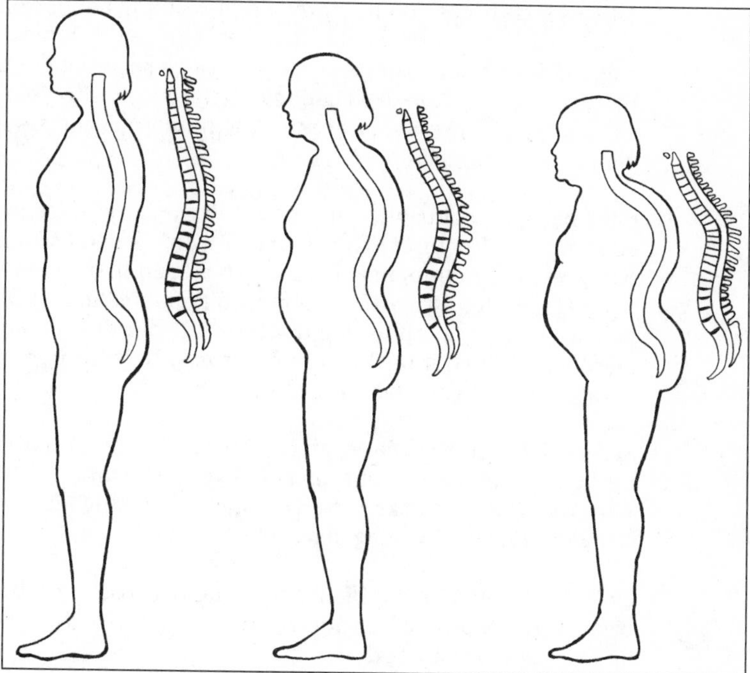

Figure 7-4: Multiple wedge fractures of the vertebrae can result in a "dowager's hump."

Compression fractures caused by osteoporosis can occur without a trauma. You don't have to fall from a ladder or be hit by a bicycle to have vertebral compression fractures.

If you have severe osteoporosis, a sneeze or cough can fracture a vertebra. Up to 30 percent of compression fractures occur when the patient is in bed! Nagging back pain may be the only symptom you have from vertebral compression fractures.

Grading vertebral fractures

The vast majority of vertebral compression fractures don't come to medical attention and are referred to as *asymptomatic* fractures. The International Osteoporosis Foundation (IOF) is encouraging radiologists to report a height loss of 20 percent in any vertebral body as a fracture so as to increase reporting and reduce ambiguity.

Although compression fractures don't result in admissions to the hospital as frequently as hip fractures, you can become just as disabled. Furthermore, the pain can be just as severe if not more so because your facture can significantly interfere with your quality of life. If your compression fractures are numerous and severe, the pain may never disappear.

Back pain and spinal deformities aren't the only consequences of compression fractures. The change in your skeletal structure can compress your abdominal organs, which can then lead to a protruding belly, constipation, decreased appetite, and weight loss. If you suffer from compression fractures in your *thoracic spine* (the middle part of your back), your lungs may become partially compressed, which can make you short of breath.

Studies have shown that each vertebral compression fracture reduces the ability of your lungs to expand by around 10 percent. With three or more fractures, you may lose enough lung capacity to cause untreatable lung disease.

Only around 10 percent of all people in their 80s are actually treated for their osteoporotic vertebral fractures. If you've lost inches, see your doctor!

The incredible shrinking person

If you're getting shorter by the year, you may assume that you have osteoporosis. Although that diagnosis is certainly possible, you may also have another disease process that is responsible for your being less able to reach the top pantry shelf.

Some other causes of height loss as you age include

- Compression fractures of vertebral bodies due to osteomalacia
- Juvenile epiphysitis (Scheuermann's disease), which affects the thoracic spine and causes the middle of your back to hunch forward
- Scoliosis (an S-shaped curvature of the spine that starts in childhood and slowly progresses through adulthood)
- Tumors involving the bones of the back
- Severe degeneration of the *discs* (the soft cartilage material in between the vertebral bodies)

So although vertebral compression fractures may result in loss of height, if you're losing inches, see your doctor to be sure you receive the proper diagnosis and treatment.

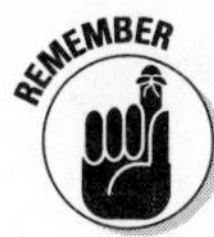

Don't forget these additional facts about compression fractures if you're a trivia buff:

- Vertebral compression fractures are the most common osteoporotic fractures. More than 700,000 occur each year in the United States.
- Approximately 25 percent of all postmenopausal women have compression fractures.
- Having compression fractures can increase your mortality rate by 15 percent. They can lead to chronic pain and severely impact your quality of life, in addition to leading to the dreaded dowager's hump.

Chapter 8

Finding (and Paying For) a Doctor to Treat Osteoporosis

In This Chapter

- Choosing the right specialist
- Finding the best doctor for *you*
- Working with your doctor
- Looking into your insurance coverage

Choosing a doctor to treat or diagnose osteoporosis can be confusing. With some diseases, the kind of doctor you choose is pretty cut and dried. For example, if you had an eye problem, you wouldn't go to a heart surgeon; you'd go to an ophthalmologist. But finding a doctor who only specializes in osteoporosis isn't as easy. In fact, you can find many types of doctors with an interest in osteoporosis in several different medical specialties.

Finding the right doctor under *any* circumstance can be a time-consuming and frustrating task. In this chapter we discuss the specialists that treat osteoporosis, a plan to find the right doctor for you, ways for you and your doctor to work together on your plan of care, and a lowdown on paying for your doctor's visits and treatment with your insurance company's help.

I Looked in the Phonebook, But I Couldn't Find Any Bone-ologists

Obstetricians deliver babies; pediatricians take care of children. But when you look in the phonebook for doctors specializing in osteoporosis, you may have no idea where to start. You certainly won't find any listings for bone-ologists. So where do you start in your search for a doctor to diagnose and treat osteoporosis?

Osteoporosis accounts for 2.5 million doctor visits and 400,000 hospital admissions yearly, and yet not one specialty is devoted strictly to osteoporosis. A family practitioner or gynecologist first sees most women for osteoporosis before possibly recommending a specialist.

Seeing your family doctor

Starting with your family doctor, who may be a family medicine specialist or an internal medicine specialist, doesn't hurt. Some internists or family medicine doctors have a special interest in osteoporosis and may be perfectly capable of handling your care. If your doctor feels you need someone whose primary practice is osteoporosis, she may send you to any number of specialists (see the next section, "Choosing a specialist").

However, one large study showed that osteoporosis is more likely to be diagnosed and treated by specialists rather than family practitioners or internists, with 96 percent of metabolic bone specialists diagnosing and treating osteoporosis in women whose osteoporosis was diagnosed by bone mineral testing as opposed to 75 percent of rheumatologists, 63 percent of endocrinologists, and 53 percent of general internists.

If your doctor doesn't want to send you to a specialist, ask her why. It may be that she is especially interested in osteoporosis and keeps up-to-date with the latest information. If so, that's fine. However, if you feel more comfortable with a specialist, tell your family doc.

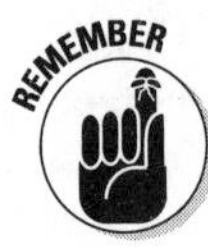

A doctor who knows your medical history well could be your best bet for treatment, as long as she keeps up with the latest treatment information and takes osteoporosis seriously.

Choosing a specialist

Many different medical specialties are available where practitioners may choose to treat patients with osteoporosis. Your primary doctor can help you decide which one of the following is best for you:

- **Rheumatologists:** Rheumatologists (your co-author Dr. O'Connor is one) diagnose and treat diseases of the bones, joints, and muscles, including autoimmune diseases such as lupus. Rheumatology is a subspecialty of internal medicine and requires board certification in both internal medicine and rheumatology.

- **Endocrinologists:** Endocrinologists treat diseases of the endocrine system, which is certainly no surprise. The endocrine system comprises the glands and hormones that control your body's metabolic activity. Endocrinologists treat diabetes, thyroid problems, and pituitary diseases. Endocrinology, like rheumatology, is a subspecialty of internal medicine.

  Endocrinologists may be especially interested in osteoporosis because endocrine problems often result in osteoporosis. Refer to Chapter 3 for a complete discussion of risk factors.

- **Geriatricians:** Geriatricians treat geriatric patients (also known as senior citizens). When are you in this category? Although most people would say "never," the accepted definition of "geriatric" is age 65 and above.

  Because osteoporosis is often, but not always, a disease of aging, many geriatricians have a special interest in treating it.

- **Gynecologists:** Because women comprise the largest group of osteoporosis patients, many gynecologists, doctors who treat women's health, also treat patients with osteoporosis. If you're a man with osteoporosis, though, you may feel a little funny sitting in the waiting room.

- **Orthopedic surgeons:** Orthopedic surgeons specialize in the treatment of bones and muscles. Some are interested in treating osteoporosis, while some aren't.

- **Physiatrists:** Physiatrists are often confused with everything from psychologists to podiatrists! Physiatrists specialize in physical medicine and rehabilitation, dealing with acute injuries as well as chronic conditions such as arthritis and osteoporosis.

Taking extra courses in bone: Metabolic bone specialists

Some doctors have taken additional training in interpreting bone mineral density tests; a doctor who has taken this type of course usually has a special interest in osteoporosis.

An international society of bone densitometry (a mouthful if there ever was one!), called the International Society of Clinical Densitometry, offers courses for physicians who are interested in discovering how to interpret bone mineral density studies. One of your authors (Dr. O'Connor) has taken such a course and therefore has special expertise in interpreting bone densitometry studies. Ask your doctor if she has taken such courses.

Some rheumatologists, endocrinologists, and orthopedic surgeons who work in academic teaching hospitals do nothing other than diagnose and treat patients with metabolic bone disease, because their research involves studying bone problems.

If your case is unusual or difficult to treat, a metabolic bone specialist is your best bet. However, most metabolic bone specialists practice in large university settings, which may be impractical to visit regularly if you live in the middle of nowhere.

You can have an initial consultation at a large university and then allow your doctor at home to follow up. This option may be good for people who don't live close to a large university but can spend a few days out of town seeing a specialist.

Preparing to Meet the Doctor

Making a list of important questions before seeing any doctor for the first time or when you're going to discuss a specific problem is always a good idea. For some reason many people's anxiety levels shoot through the roof when visiting the doctor's office, often causing them to forget why they came in. Maybe the antiseptic smell or the white lab coats do it, but something about the whole environment can be frightening. Be prepared and make a list so you don't forget.

Everyone's list will be a little different, but use the following basic questions to get started:

- Do you treat many patients with osteoporosis?
- What kind of diagnostic tests do you usually conduct?
- Will you call me when you get the results, or do I need a follow-up appointment?
- How can I reach you if I have questions?
- Will my insurance pay for the tests to be done?
- What is your background in treating osteoporosis? Have you taken additional training to treat it?

You may not be comfortable asking the doctor questions, because you were raised not to question the doctor. Don't worry about asking the doctor for clarification. Most doctors today are interested in educating their patients and want you to ask questions about anything that isn't clear to you. So ask away! And if your doctor doesn't feel that way, she may not be the right doctor for you!

Before you even walk in the door, you can ask the office staff the following questions:

- What medical school did the physician attend?
- Where did the physician receive her postgraduate training?
- Is the physician board certified?
- Does the physician's office have its own bone density equipment?
- With what hospitals is the physician affiliated? Some insurance companies have this data available on their Web sites. The Web might list the medical schools of the physicians who participate in their network, for example.

Getting ready for your first appointment

Before you go for your first appointment, put together a manila folder of "must have's," so you don't forget anything. Make sure to put the following items in the folder:

- Your list of questions (See "Preparing to Meet the Doctor" earlier in this chapter.)
- Your medical records, including blood tests done within the last two years and consultations with other physicians
- The scans from your Dual Energy X-ray Absorptiometry (DXA scan), a specific type of test that measures your bone mineral density (see Chapter 9 for more on the DXA scan)
- Any X-rays (the actual X-rays, not just the reports)
- A list of drugs you're taking for your osteoporosis, as well as a list of all other medications and vitamins you take with dosages, including any over-the-counter (OTC) medications

- A list of all other health issues you have, because they may affect your doctor's recommendations
- A list of your other doctors' names and phone numbers just in case your doctor wants to speak with them to coordinate your care

Making sure you've found Dr. Right

Finding the right doctor isn't always easy. Even if the doctor you're seeing has the best reputation in town, he may not be right for you if:

- He makes you feel uncomfortable asking questions.
- He doesn't answer your questions to your satisfaction.
- He doesn't call you back within a reasonable time when you have concerns.

You may need more than one visit to figure out whether your new doctor is right for you. Your first visit may be awkward for a number of reasons: you're nervous, the doctor is having a bad day, the office seems disorganized with long waiting times, or the front-desk staff is unfriendly. Don't let one bad experience scare you away, *if* you feel comfortable with the doctor otherwise.

Team Tactics: Setting Up a Care Plan with Your Doctor

When making a plan for treating osteoporosis, you need to work closely with your doctor. The days of doctors just telling you what to do and you doing it, without understanding why or for how long, are long gone. Most doctors today are well aware that patients want and have a right to be involved in their own care and to understand what medications they're taking and why.

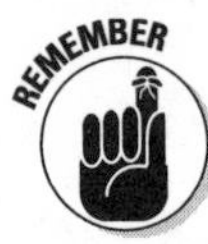

The first step in treatment is diagnosis. Ask your doctor if she plans to do a DXA scan (see Chapter 9 for the full details about the scan) to assess your baseline bone density. If she says no, ask why! Determining whether your treatment is helpful if you don't know where you started from, as a basis for comparison, is difficult. Ask how often she wants to do scans; make sure your insurance will pay for scans at the timeframe she recommends. (See "Getting the Most Out of Your Insurance Plan" later in this chapter for important insurance info.)

After you have a diagnosis, formulate a treatment plan with your doctor. Every treatment plan has several facets to consider:

- **Prognosis:** How is osteoporosis likely to affect me? Your family history and your current health history, including medication, influence your prognosis.
- **Medications:** Your treatment plan may include medication to prevent osteoporosis or slow bone loss, as well as supplements such as calcium and vitamin D. (See Chapter 10 for more on medications and osteoporosis.)

Make sure you discuss with your doctor other medications (including all OTC meds, vitamins, and supplements) you're taking for other medical conditions. She needs to know the specific drugs and dosages to make sure she doesn't prescribe something for your osteoporosis that interacts with your other medication.

- **Dietary recommendations:** Your doctor can suggest ideas for increasing calcium and other necessary nutrients in your diet. (See Chapter 5 for more on osteoporosis and diet.)
- **Exercise plan:** An exercise plan doesn't have to mean spending hours at the gym. Simple weight training or just increasing your normal physical activity can all be part of your exercise plan. (See Chapter 6 for more on exercise and osteoporosis.)
- **Reassessment:** You may need to see your doctor regularly to gauge whether or not your current treatments are effective. A plan isn't worth anything if it isn't getting the desired results.

Your doctor may also be able to supply you with a list of support groups for osteoporosis sufferers in your area. Many local hospitals run monthly support meetings where you can connect with people who can relate to what you're going through — and possibly make some new friends, too.

Depression is common in people with chronic illness. Don't be afraid to mention to your doctor — or your family members, for that matter — that you're struggling with depression. Your doctor may be able to refer you to a therapist specially trained in the area of aging, or to a support group. The worst thing you can do when you're hurting emotionally is to hide it — resources are available to help you through tough emotional times.

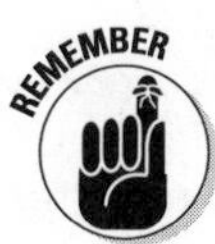

Your physician may need to collect more data before making a decision about your treatment, so don't be upset if she wants to see you again before giving out medications or specific plans. Making sure your doctor has all the pertinent information before deciding on a treatment is in your best interest.

Being honest with your doctor

Some people sometimes tell their doctor whatever it is he wants to hear, even if they know perfectly well they're not going to follow his recommendations. Obviously, doing so isn't in your best interest!

Even if you think your doctor will be angry with you, don't tell him you're willing to do something you know perfectly well you won't! Be completely honest and upfront about your personal needs and limitations. And if you find yourself unable to be honest with your doctor, ask yourself why. Does he get upset when you question him, or does he refuse to discuss alternatives? It may be time to find another doctor!

Discussing your diet and exercise habits

Diet and exercise are two prime areas that seem most likely to bring out the fibber in people, but they're certainly not the only two. Lifestyle changes such as quitting smoking or drinking aren't too far behind.

Many people don't like to admit to their doctor that, despite their heartfelt promises in the office, they probably aren't going to start going to the gym four times a week — at least, not for more than a week or two! And your intention to eliminate coffee and soda from your diet and to add three cups of cottage cheese a day — well, are you seriously going to do it? Even more important, are you going to tell your doctor you *did* do it at your next visit?

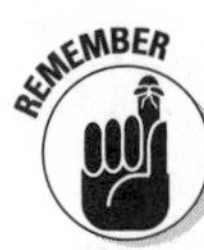

Even at the risk of feeling like you're letting your doctor down, be honest about your shortcomings. If you admit you're unlikely to head for the gym in January, your doctor may come up with a more practical plan — one that lets you exercise in your own home. If the thought of putting on a leotard — or even sweats — at the local Muscle Busters gym has you hiding behind the couch, admit that you're too embarrassed to set foot in a gym staffed with and populated by twenty-somethings. Your doctor may know of exercise programs catering to seniors, or programs designed for people who haven't exercised in a while.

If you didn't make all these changes but tell your doctor you did, he may be baffled at your lack of response. Or, being a fairly astute person, he may surmise that you're not being entirely truthful with him!

The same policy of telling the truth at all costs applies to lifestyle changes. If you're still smoking, admit it and ask for help in quitting or at least cutting down. If you hate cottage cheese, ask for some suggestions for other calcium-rich foods.

Discussing medication

Don't lie about taking your medication. If you stopped taking it two months ago because it upset your stomach, tell your doctor. Another brand or type of medication may work fine, or he may suggest a different way for you to take your medication to minimize upset.

But if your doctor thinks you're still taking your medication, he may be baffled by your lack of response, not realizing that your lack of response is related to your lack of taking your medicine. He may then prescribe a stronger medication or higher dose, which could be unnecessary or even harmful to you.

Being honest with yourself

Being honest with yourself is just another part of being honest with your doctor. You probably know yourself pretty well, and you know what you are and aren't going to do, even in the name of being healthier. You can't admit to your doctor that you're never going to follow an exercise program if you don't first admit it to yourself!

The problem with lying to yourself is that you cheat yourself out of possible alternatives. If you promise yourself that you're going to go to the gym faithfully in March, you may drift into April before admitting that you missed the boat. If you would have admitted in February that going to the gym would never be part of your after-work routine, you could have made an alternate plan, such as walking three times a week during your lunch hour in the mall. Yes, you may have stopped at the winter clearance sales racks once or twice a week, but you certainly would have gotten more exercise than you did by promising yourself you'd get to the gym and never getting there.

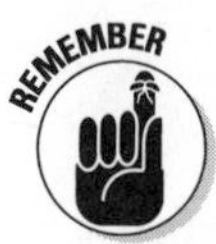

The only person who suffers the consequences of deceiving yourself — or your doctor — is *you*. Be honest about what you can and can't do so you can maximize your treatment plan within your own limitations.

Keeping in touch after your visit

Your doctor will most likely suggest a follow-up appointment in a month or two to check on your progress. Keep your follow-up appointments! As busy as you may be, you can't substitute anything for a face-to-face visit.

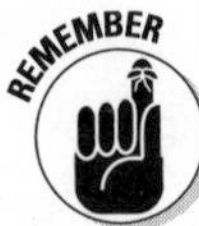

Although you may be tempted just to phone in a report, telephone consultations never provide adequate care. Most physicians are hurried and can't provide the same attention to detail over the telephone as they can when you're in the office.

Getting the Most Out of Your Insurance Plan

You may have a love-hate relationship with your insurance provider. On one hand, knowing you're protected against outrageous bills in case of illness is good. On the other hand, how can you make heads or tails out of what your policy covers and what it doesn't cover?

Because hundreds, if not thousands, of variations of policies are available on what health insurers will and won't pay, we really can't tell you what your insurance will cover when it comes to osteoporosis testing and visits. If you're covered by insurance, read your insurance manuals (you know, the 500-page books you tossed in a closet somewhere) thoroughly to see what coverage you have and if you need referrals from your primary care physician. You may also need to call your company representatives for clarification of the rules, if they seem unclear.

Calling back more than once may be worthwhile if the first person you speak to doesn't seem sure about your coverage, or if her advice seems to contradict what's in the book. The next person you speak with may give more satisfactory answers. If she does, write down her name and keep detailed notes about the conversation!

Although insurance companies differ, we can give you the basic guidelines for Medicare coverage, as well as a summary of laws passed by different states about osteoporosis.

According to the National Osteoporosis Foundation (NOF), Medicare will pay for a DXA scan every two years if you're in one of the following groups:

- An estrogen-deficient woman, as defined by her doctor
- An individual with vertebral deformities, such as scoliosis
- An individual on long-term corticosteroid therapy
- An individual with primary hyperparathyroidism
- An individual being monitored to assess response of efficacy of a FDA-approved osteoporosis drug therapy

People who are or will be taking the equivalent of 7.5 mg a day of prednisone, a corticosteroid, may be able to have DXA scans more frequently than every two years.

Seven states, California, Florida, Louisiana, Maryland, North Carolina, Oklahoma, and Texas, have mandated private insurance coverage for osteoporosis-related diagnostic testing and treatment. Some, such as Kentucky, require insurers to offer baseline bone density testing starting at age 35. Others, like Maryland, require that testing requested by a healthcare provider be covered.

Three other states — Georgia, Kentucky, and Tennessee — have laws that require plans to offer coverage for osteoporosis-related testing and treatment. It may cost you extra to add it to your insurance plan, however. Thirty-three states have laws relating to osteoporosis; some sponsor osteoporosis-awareness programs, while others provide funding for testing for low income and uninsured women.

For a thorough rundown of state-by-state coverage and programs relating to osteoporosis, check out `www.ncsl.org`. You can also check out the appendix in this book for a state-by-state list of programs. To look at Medicare coverage, go to `http://medicare.gov/coverage/home/asp`.

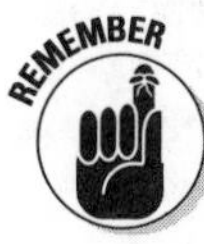

If you're unemployed and below a certain income, you can apply for medical assistance from your state. Each state has different requirements. A financial counselor at a hospital or social worker has the skills and knowledge to assist with this problem. Don't avoid seeking care because of the lack of insurance, because the system may have a way to help you.

Eeny meeny miney moe — did I choose an HMO?

Insurance companies just love acronyms and abbreviations. Have you ever called to find one to find about coverage and had to answer the question "Is your plan a PPO, POS, or an HMO?" This question leaves you scrambling to find a magnifying glass to read the small print on the back of the card, because you have no idea what you are or what those initials mean.

First, a few definitions:

- HMO stands for health maintenance organization. Many people with osteoporosis have a health plan that is an HMO. Generally, if you have an HMO, referrals are required for seeing specialists, obtaining X-rays, and for physical therapy.

- PPO stands for Preferred Provider Organization. In a PPO, you aren't required to get referrals, but you must see a physician who is in your network.
- POS stands for Point of Service. POS is the least restrictive, but in some cases, you might still need to see network providers.

Regardless of the type of health insurance, your plan may decide that certain treatment is medically unnecessary and consequently may deny coverage of certain treatment.

The best way to avoid this kind of aggravation is to know your coverage ahead of time. First, know what services are covered. Second, understand your specific plan's rules. For example, are referrals necessary? If you use an HMO, find out if you need a referral for laboratory testing and X-rays.

Most health plans have an (usually large) section called "exclusions and limitations." This section tells you what your insurance won't pay for. Find out the services that your plan doesn't cover. Physical therapy sections are especially important if you have osteoporosis.

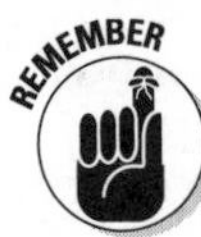

Know which hospitals are covered in your health plan in case you require admission to a hospital, or even an emergency visit. If you go to a hospital not covered in your plan, you may spend weeks on the phone arguing to get your visit paid for.

What if you have a disagreement with your insurance company? For example, you've read your manual from cover to cover and believe that a certain service is covered, but the payment is denied. You can appeal! The Kaiser Family Foundation has published a 73-page document that is available online at `www.kff.org/insurance/index.cfm`, which details exactly how to appeal. The site also includes a worksheet so that you can begin to understand your coverage.

If you need to file an appeal, follow these steps:

1. **Contact the plan's customer relations department.**

   Be sure to take notes regarding every phone call, including whom you spoke with, the date, and time.

2. **If it still isn't resolved, make a formal appeal in writing to your plan.**

   Send the letter certified mail and keep a copy for your records.

3. **If you still don't get a resolution, you can proceed with another level of appeal called an *external appeal.***

   Because state governments handle most laws related to health insurance companies, the process of external reviews varies.

Going out of network

If your plan uses *capitation,* you may be restricted in terms of where you go for laboratory testing, radiographs, and physical therapy. In other words, if you want your insurance to pay, you need to stay "in network" and use the lab the insurance sends you to.

However, your primary care doctor can often give you an "out of network" referral if she feels it's important for you to see a specific doctor not in your network. Some insurance plans have a higher *co-pay,* an amount you pay upfront at the time of the visit, if you go out of network.

Getting your drugs covered

Until recently, Medicare didn't provide any prescription coverage. In 2003, the Medicare Modernization Act was enacted. It provides some level of coverage for medications related to bone health.

Some plans, for reasons of their own making, cover one brand name of drug and not another, so make sure your doctor orders the one that's covered, unless she has a specific reason for using a certain brand. Most prescription plans don't cover multivitamins or calcium supplements.

Chapter 9

Testing Your Bones

In This Chapter

- Understanding how bone density testing works
- Determining who needs bone density testing
- Testing your bones in other ways
- Interpreting your test results
- Figuring out how often to get tested

You may have heard people talk about bone density tests without really having any idea what they are. But you think maybe you need one, because everyone else in your book club has, and you want to know what you're talking about when you make your appointment.

Obviously, the test has something to do with your bones, the density of your bones, and minerals. You may have no idea whether it's a blood test, an X-ray, or an exercise test.

Cheer up. In this chapter, we thoroughly educate you on the ins and outs of bone density testing, which is sometimes called *bone densitometry,* a word only your doctor will be able to correctly pronounce.

After you read this chapter, you'll be able to discuss your DXA (pronounced dexa) and a whole alphabet of initials with the best of them. Bone density measurements also go by several other terms, including DeXA, DXA (DXA is the preferred abbreviation, but either abbreviation is used), bone mineral density testing, and bone densitometry. If your doctor uses one of these terms, just know she wants you to get your bone density measured.

What's Bone Density Testing, Anyway?

Bone density testing, or *bone densitometry* is a radiological way to measure your bone density. Bone density measures the strength of your bones and helps predict the chance that you'll sustain a bone fracture due to osteoporosis. The lower your bone density, the more likely you are to fracture a bone even after a slight injury.

Bone density can be measured by several different tests, which we review in the next section. A bone density test can tell you how your bone mass and strength stack up against others in your age group. The overall accuracy of bone mineral density tests is 85 to 99 percent.

Are you wondering why these specialized tests are even necessary? Why not just get an X-ray and be on your merry way? Standard X-rays aren't a good way to measure bone density because your doctor can't see or detect any bone loss on the X-ray until you've lost at least 30 percent of your bone mass. Clearly you and your doctor need to know about bone loss long before you lose that much.

Deciding When to Have a Bone Density Test

The International Society of Densitometry has made certain recommendations for bone density testing (your co-author Dr. O'Connor endorses these recommendations). The following people need a bone density test:

- All women aged 65 and older
- Postmenopausal women under age 65 with risk factors such as
    - Smoking
    - Weight less than 126 pounds
    - Family history of osteoporosis
- All men aged 70 and older
- Any adults with a history of a fragility fracture (including hip, wrist, and spinal fracture with minimal trauma)

- Adults with a disease or condition associated with low bone mass or bone loss (see Chapter 3)
- Adults taking medications associated with low bone mass or bone loss (see Chapter 3)
- Anyone being considered for treatment
- Anyone being treated with drugs for osteoporosis to monitor treatment effect
- Anyone not receiving therapy where evidence of bone loss would lead to treatment, such as a patient with previously diagnosed osteopenia now stopping estrogen treatment
- All patients with evidence of reduced bone density on regular skeletal X-rays

The National Osteoporosis Foundation (NOF) also has recommendations about when to have a bone density test:

- All women age 65 and older
- Postmenopausal women under age 65 with
  - Family history of osteoporosis
  - Personal history of low-trauma fracture after age 45
  - Current cigarette smoker
  - Low body weight (less than 127 pounds)
- Other clinical indications include
  - Low-trauma fractures as an adult
  - Hyperthyroidism
  - Hyperparathyroidism
  - Rheumatoid arthritis
  - Vitamin D deficiency
  - Diseases that cause poor intestinal absorption such as sprue (see Chapter 3 for a list)
- Use of medications that cause bone loss include
  - Excessive doses of corticosteroids
  - Medications that block sex hormone production
  - Medications used to treat seizures
  - Thyroid hormone medications

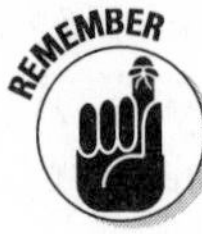

Medicare covers your bone density test every two years if you're postmenopausal. (Medicare also covers other diagnoses.) (Check out Chapter 8, which discusses Medicare and private insurance coverage.) You can't have a bone density test unless your physician orders the test with a diagnosis listed on your prescription.

DXA, SXA, PDXA, and More — Understanding This Alphabet Soup

Although you may assume that a bone density test is a bone density test is a bone density test, and who cares what kind you have, however, it really does pay to know what the different tests accomplish.

Deciphering DXA

When people talk about having a bone density test, the Dual Energy X-Ray Absorptiometry (DXA) is usually the test they're having. The DXA scan, often considered the gold standard for bone mineral density tests, is the most widely available test and the one most insurance companies cover.

A DXA scan (see Figure 9-1) typically measures the density of your lower spine and your left hip. Many DXA scanners can also measure the strength of your wrist bone. Taking your wrist's measurement is especially important if your doctor or the technician can't measure the density of your spine or hip. Most doctors prefer to have at least two different sites studied.

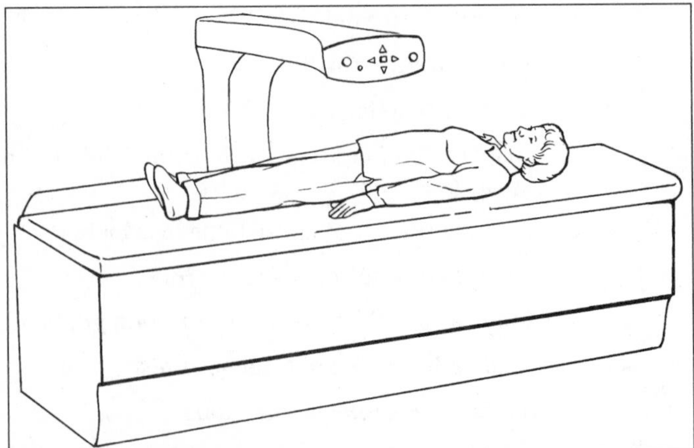

Figure 9-1: A woman getting a DXA.

A DXA scan is quite accurate, absolutely painless, and requires no advance preparation. You don't have to fast, receive any injections or sedation, take any kind of medication, or even memorize your multiplication tables before the test. The only preparation is not to take calcium tablets the day before and the day of the procedure. You want to avoid the calcium supplements because they can artificially increase the bone density in your spine if they're still in your intestine.

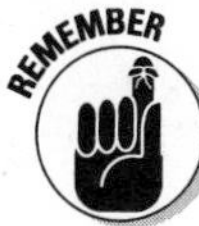

You can keep your clothes on during the examination, as long you don't wear anything with metal buttons or zippers. You may be asked to remove metal jewelry. (The metal can increase bone density dramatically, which can skew the results.)

You lie on an exam table for a DXA scan, and the test takes only a short time to complete, less than 15 minutes or so. A DXA scan does subject you to a dose of radiation, but the amount is small — less than what you'd receive during a chest X-ray (about 1/30th of the dose). The scan directs X-rays from two different sources (hence the name "Dual Energy") at your bone in an alternating pattern.

There is almost no scatter of radiation either, so the room doesn't require shielding. You may find DXA machines in your doctor's office, which is the most commonly performed type of test.

Settling for SXA

The SXA test (which stands for Single Energy X-Ray Absorptiometry) measures the bone density in the forearm or heel. The SXA has several main disadvantages compared to the DXA scan including:

- The part being tested has to be submersed in water.
- The test also measures only bone sites that are far from the spine and hip. Bone density readings in the heel may not correlate with bone density readings in your back.
- The SXA test may not be as accurate.
- It takes longer to complete.

Meanwhile, the advantages of the test include the following:

- The equipment is portable.
- The cost is low.

Pondering PDXA

Peripheral Dual Energy X-Ray Absorptiometry (PDXA) measures only peripheral sites, such as the wrist, heel, or finger, and it takes less time to complete than the SXA. The equipment, like the SXA, is portable, but the cost is higher than the SXA.

The PDXA delivers a very low radiation dose, and like the DXA, it has high resolution and a high degree of accuracy.

Looking at the RA

Radiographic Absorptiometry (RA), otherwise known as *photodensitometry,* has the advantage of using standard X-ray equipment, but it requires specialized equipment that scans film at high resolution. Then your doctor uses specialized software to calculate bone volume, bone density, and cortical thickness. It also delivers a minimal dose of radiation.

On the downside, it measures the strength of bone in only your fingers, and doctors and researchers have yet to determine the correlation of this reading with density elsewhere in the body.

Questioning pQCT

Peripheral Quantitative Computed Tomography (pQCT) is a very accurate test done by using a traditional CAT scanner with specialized software. This test, which is primarily utilized in research, is very accurate but expensive, and it results in a higher exposure to radiation. It also takes longer to obtain the scan.

The pQCT is the only test that can measure *cortical bone* (the outer shell) and *trabecular bone* (the inner honeycomb layer) in the forearm. (See Chapter 2 for the lowdown on bones.)

Testing Bones in Other Ways

The tests previously mentioned in this chapter all use radiation, although in low amounts, to measure bone mineral density. Three other tests are available that can look at your bones without radiation: ultrasound and blood and urine tests.

Bone turnover (no cherry or blueberry) markers

Recent exciting research has shown that high levels of resorption markers in your blood or urine may predict the development of hip fracture. (See Chapter 2.) At this point in time, these biochemical markers are measured under very special circumstances or in complex cases.

Just in case you really want to know what resorption and formation markers are, here are the official technical descriptions:

- **Resorption markers:** As bone is resorbed, collagen is broken down into fragments. The resorption markers measure these breakdown products. You may have heard of the names of these tests; examples are N teleopeptide (NTX) and C teleopeptide (CTX).
- **Formation markers:** These markers measure certain proteins that are made and released into the blood during the process of bone formation. The names of these markers are osteocalcin and bone specific alkaline phosphatase (BSAP).

Ultrasound tests

Taking an ultrasound of your heel is the second most common way of evaluating for osteoporosis, after the DXA scan. It's simple and inexpensive, but it probably isn't as accurate as the DXA scan.

Blood and urine tests

Researchers and doctors are developing new blood and urine tests that attempt to measure the rate of bone turnover. In other words, exactly what is the balance of bone formation and bone resorption (breakdown) in you?

Doctors refer to these tests as "biochemical markers of bone turnover." These markers are more useful for monitoring the treatment and progress of osteoporosis and not for measuring bone mass.

Interpreting the Results of Your DXA

Bone density scans can be a confusing jumble of T-scores and Z-scores, and plus and minus signs, unless someone explains how to interpret them. (Today is your lucky day. We're here to help you!)

Knowing your T-score

Your *T-score* compares your bone mineral density, with the young normal average bone mineral density and expresses the difference as a standard deviation score. If you're shaking your head, rest assured that we explain these scores more in-depth in this section.

You figure your T-score with the following formula:

> T-score = (Patient's bone mineral density – Young Normal Mean) divided by
>
> Standard Deviation of Young Normal Mean

To explain in simpler words, your T-score is your bone mineral density compared to the average (mean) score of young adults (ages 25 to 35). These young adults have your same gender and ethnicity. The difference between the two is called a "standard deviation" abbreviated SD.

The SD is your T-score, which can be either a plus or minus number. If your T-score is zero, then your bone density is exactly the same as the average value of women (or men) of the population of young women of your race.

If your T-score is greater than zero, for example, +1, then your bone density is 1 standard deviation greater than the average young population. In contrast, a T-score less than 0, for example, –1, means that your bone density is less than the average of younger women. The lower the T-score, the lower your bone density compared to younger women.

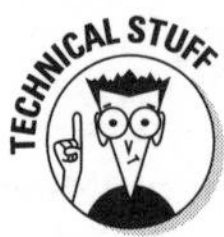

Another way of looking at bone density is to look at the actual value of the measurement in grams per area or grams per centimeters squared. This number is an actual measurement of density and your doctor can monitor it.

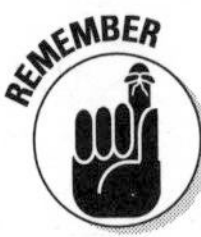

Your risk of fracture is related to your T-score. Based upon your T-score, your doctor can use special tables to predict your risk of future fracture at each site and your age. To explain it another way, your risk of fracture doubles every time your T-score drops by 1.0. Your doctor can also use your T-score to predict the chance you might have a fracture over the next ten years.

Your doctor uses the T-score and an assessment of your other risk factors for osteoporosis (see Chapter 3 for the different risk factors) and then decides if you need treatment for prevention of further bone loss. Your T-scores may differ at different sites of your body because bone may lose its strength at different rates.

To make T-scores a little easier to understand, Table 9-1 explains the break points between normal bone, osteopenia, and osteoporosis, based on definitions from the World Health Organization (WHO).

Table 9-1 WHO Definitions of Osteoporosis Based on Bone Density T-scores

Bone Mineral density	***T-score***
Normal	1 standard deviation (SD) or less below the young adult reference range (–1)
Low bone mass (osteopenia)	1 to 2.5 SDs below the young adult reference range (–1 to –2.5)
Osteoporosis	2.5 or more SDs below the young adult reference range (–2.5 or less)
Severe osteoporosis	2.5 or more SDs below the young adult reference range (–2.5 or less) and the presence of one or more bone fractures

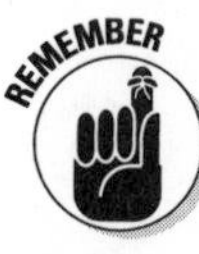

A T-score doesn't tell your doctor about the cause of your low bone density. You may have osteomalacia (see Chapter 1), which is another important cause of low bone strength and isn't technically the same condition as osteoporosis. If you have a very low T-score, then in all likelihood your primary care doctor will refer you to a specialist who can try to determine the reason why your bone strength is so much lower than the average.

What if your T-score is in the normal range, yet you suffer a fragility fracture (see Chapter 7 for more about fragility fractures)? If this happens, you need to see a bone specialist.

Catching the Z's

Now, you may think comparing your bone density with that of a 25-to-35-year-old is unfair, especially if you're on the far side of 50. Someone must have agreed with you on that point, because another score, called the Z-score, compares your results to other people your same age, gender, height, and weight.

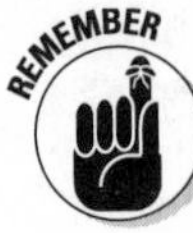

A negative number in the Z-score isn't good, because it means your bones are thinner than those of your contemporaries who have similar height, weight, age, and gender. A positive number means you have less chance of fracture than others in your demographically similar group.

Z-scores are more useful in measuring bone density in children, because you want to compare bone density to other children of the same age.

Interpreting all these numbers

Although you may think it's unfair, your doctor will use the lowest, or worst score you got as your bone mineral density score, which means that if your hips aren't bad but your spine is, the spine number is the one she's going to use.

Your doctor will also need to look at your overall health as part of your evaluation, because some diseases can result in a lower than normal bone mineral density, even if you don't have osteoporosis. Some of the diseases that can lower your bone mineral density are

- Ankylosing spondylitis
- Cushing disease
- Hyperparathyroidism
- Hyperthyroidism
- Multiple myeloma
- Premature menopause
- Rheumatoid arthritis
- Rickets
- Vitamin D deficiency

See Chapter 3 for more information about these specific diseases and how they affect your bone density.

Knowing How Often You Need a Bone Density Test

One bone density test in your lifetime isn't always enough. In fact, your doctor may ask you to have tests done every year or so if you fall into certain categories, as we outline in this section.

For example, your doctor may prescribe serial bone mineral testing to monitor your response to treatment, or to monitor you if you're at risk for rapid bone loss, such as if you take high doses of corticosteroids.

The International Society of Bone Densitometry recommends:

> "Repeating bone density typically one year after initiation or change of therapy with longer intervals once therapeutic effect is established. In conditions associated with rapid bone loss, such as glucocorticoid therapy, more often might be appropriate."

However, the changes in bone density after one year on treatment are very slight, perhaps beyond the detection of bone density readings. If you experienced a dramatic decline in bone density after one year (for example, greater than 5 percent), your doctor perhaps may change the therapy. However, not many people have such a decline. People on high doses of corticosteroids may be in this category.

Repeating your DXA scan every two years is an approach that many experts in the field take. Your doctor will compare bone mineral densities from year to year. Make sure you or you doctor don't compare T-scores.

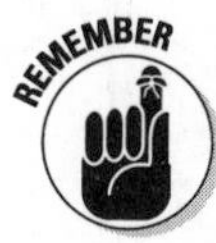

Also, bone mineral densities from different manufacturers aren't readily comparable. Therefore if you return to the same radiological unit year after year for your DXA scan, make sure the equipment has the same manufacturer.

Chapter 10

Taking Prescription Drugs for Osteoporosis

In This Chapter

- Glancing at the available drugs
- Understanding the new "miracle" drugs for osteoporosis
- Looking at hormone replacement therapy (the good and the bad)
- Assessing the old standby drugs
- Deciding to use preventive drugs
- Watching the horizon: What's new for the future?

Some days you may feel a bit like Alice in Wonderland, taking "one pill that makes you taller, one that makes you small, and even one that doesn't do anything at all." It's nice to think that any ill can be cured with the right drug, and certainly some nearly miraculous new osteoporosis drugs are available on the market.

However, when choosing medication, "one size fits all" is a misnomer. In this chapter, we look at the different medications available for osteoporosis, who they're likely to benefit, and how to determine what's right for you. We also include a useful table that gives you a quick once-over about the available drugs by generic and brand names.

Sorting Out the Different Types of Drug Treatment

Maybe you're sitting around one day at the book club, getting a little off topic discussing the medicines your doctor has you on for osteoporosis. "Oh, my doctor said Fosamax is the best," says one friend, while another shakes her head. "Oh, no, my doctor said I have to take Evista." Meanwhile you're thinking that your doctor wants you to take injections; why can't you just take pills like your friends?

If you've ever wondered why your doctor has chosen a certain medication for you to treat your osteoporosis, take heart. We're here to help you sort out the different categories of drugs to treat osteoporosis and to explain why your doctor may choose one over the other. Osteoporosis is a problem with various causes, and the treatment from individual to individual varies depending upon the cause of the problem.

To help you, we first list the common categories of drugs and the brand names they're known by (see Table 10-1).

Table 10-1 Keeping the Drugs Straight

Generic Name	***Brand Name***
Bisphosphonates (diphosphonates)	
Alendronate	Fosamax
Risedronate	Actonel
Ibandronate sodium	Boniva
Pamidronate	Aredia
Zoledronic acid	Zometa
Etidronate (older medication)	
Other Medications	
Calcitonin	Miacalcin
Raloxifene	Evista
Teriparatide (rhPTH)	Forteo
Tibolone**	Livial
Strontium**	Protelos
Hormone Replacement	
Conjugated estrogen	Cenestin
Premarin	
Estradiol	Estrace

Generic Name	*Brand Name*
Esterified estrogen	Estratab
Menest	
Estreopipate	Ogen
Testosterone gel	Androgel

*** not yet available in the United States*

Looking at Bisphosphonates for Building Up Bone

Bones are like a bank; your bone "balance" stays healthy as long as you're not taking out more than you put in. That analogy may be a little simplistic (see Chapter 2 for the more involved detail of bone buildup and breakdown) but in essence, bone strength depends upon the balance between the bone cells that build bone versus those cells that break down bone.

Researchers have used the "bone strength equals bone buildup minus bone loss" formula to develop drugs that prevent and treat bone loss. Drugs that slow down bone breakdown are referred to as antiresorptive drugs. The wonderful part of antiresorptive drugs is that not only do they build bone density, but they also actually reduce the frequency of bone fracture.

Bisphosphonates are a type of antiresorptive drug that inhibits bone removal by the osteoclasts (see Chapter 2 for more on osteoclasts). Taking bisphosphonates can increase bone density in both the hip (by 3 percent) and lumbar spine (by 5 percent). Changes in bone density can be seen in the first year of treatment. Fracture rates are reduced by 50 percent.

Using alendronate, ibandronate, and risedronate

The most commonly used antiresorptive drugs belong to a class of compounds referred to as bisphosphonates, also called diphosphonates. Three oral bisphosphonates are approved in the United States for both prevention and treatment of osteoporosis:

- Alendronate (Fosamax)
- Ibandronate (Boniva) (the newest drug, it may be difficult to find)
- Risedronate (Actonel)

All bisphosphonates bind to *osteoclasts* (cells that break down bone) and slow their ability to resorb bone. The drugs differ somewhat in their chemical makeup, but all are antiresorptive drugs, with alendronate being the first developed.

You may find that you tolerate one drug better than the other. For example, alendronate may cause you more difficulty with stomach irritation, and risedronate may not. Ibandronate may be your choice because it only needs to be taken once a month. All the bisphosphonates vary in their side effects and their dosing regimens. People also respond to different drugs differently, so if you start with one and have side effects, don't hesitate to tell your doctor!

You may hear alendronate, ibandronate, and risedronate called "diphosphonates" instead of "bisphosphonates." A diphosphonate is the same thing as a bisphosphonate; just chalk it up to the idiosyncrasies of the scientific world to have two words (long ones, at that) for the same thing. The prefix bis- and di- both refer to the word "two." These drugs contain two phosphonate groups attached to one carbon atom. This particular structure is responsible for the strong binding of the drug to osteoclasts.

Deciding when to treat with bisphosphonates

When is it time to start bisphosphonates? When everyone else in your bridge group is on them? When your children keep hounding you about taking something for your bones? No.

Your doctor makes the final determination of when to start medications for osteoporosis, but she usually follows these guidelines for starting treatment:

- T-score is less than 2.5. (A *T-score* is the number of standard deviations the bone mineral density measurement is above or below the young normal mean bone mineral density. In other words, your T-score is your score compared to that of young adults. See Chapter 9 for the complete lowdown on T-scores.)

- T-score is less than 2.0 with multiple risk factors, such as corticosteroid use and low body mass index (BMI). (See Chapter 3 for more on risk factors.)
- T-score is less than 1.5 and you're taking drugs that cause rapid bone loss, such as corticosteroids and phenobarbitol. (See Chapter 3 for drugs that cause bone loss.)
- Menopausal status is a factor because rapid bone loss can occur in menopause due to a decrease in estrogen. (See Chapter 3 for more information about menopause's effects on osteoporosis.)

Who shouldn't take bisphosphonates?

Not everyone is a good candidate for taking bisphosphonates. Your doctor may decide not to give you bisphosphonates if you have any of the following conditions:

- Esophageal strictures
- Kidney disease
- Severe gastroesophageal reflux
- Vitamin D deficiency

Some people develop side effects that are intolerable, such as stomach irritation, or muscle and joint pain. Sometimes switching from one bisphosphonate to another may help. Among the newer bisphosphonatelike drugs, there is no clear advantage of one medication versus another in preventing fractures.

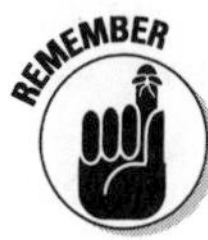

Taking bisphosphonates with adequate amounts of calcium and vitamin D is critical. You need 1,500 mg of calcium daily and 400 to 800 International Units (IU) of vitamin D daily. Check with your doctor to find out the right amount for you.

Remember that over-the-counter medications, including herbs and homeopathic remedies, are still drugs. Inform your doctor of all medications you take so she can monitor them.

Taking bisphosphonates correctly

Some bisphosphonates can be given in either daily or weekly doses as a preventive. For risedronate (Actonel), the dose is 5 mg daily or 35 mg once a week. Doctors often prescribe alendronate

(Fosamax) in a higher dose (10 mg daily or 70 mg once a week). The Food and Drug Administration (FDA) approved ibandronate (Boniva) in 2005 to be taken once a month.

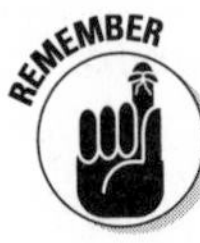

All bisphosphonates need to be taken first thing in the morning with eight ounces of water. Don't eat or drink anything else for 30 minutes after taking your medication. You need to remain upright for about 30 minutes — no sneaking back to bed for a quick nap — to help decrease stomach irritation after taking your medication.

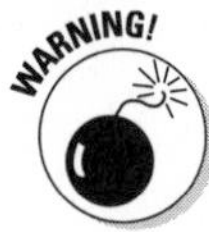

These drugs are absorbed slowly from the gastrointestinal tract. They can cause an irritation of the esophagus (a chemical esophagitis). You must use them with caution if you have any problems with your esophagus. Taking them with water is important because water doesn't compete with the drugs' absorption in the stomach; juice or other foods interfere with absorption.

The Estrogen Replacement Controversy

Bisphosphonates, or antiresorptive drugs, only act on bone tissue; they don't have an effect elsewhere in your body. Estrogen and other sex hormones, such as testosterone, on the other hand, have many effects on your body rather than acting just on bone.

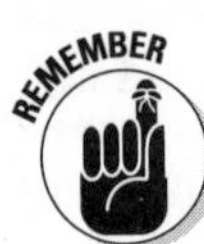

Estrogen prevents and treats osteoporosis by slowing down bone resorption. Estrogen also alleviates the symptoms of menopause, which can be terribly disabling. These symptoms include insomnia, hot flashes, and vaginal dryness. Before the development of alendronate (Fosamax), estrogens were the most commonly used drugs used for treatment of osteoporosis. Your doctor may recommend estrogen therapy if you can't tolerate the side effects of bisphosphonates or if she thinks you'll benefit in other ways, such as relief from postmenopausal symptoms, from estrogen replacement.

The FDA first approved estrogen replacement therapy for treatment of osteoporosis in 1972. However, researchers found that estrogen taken without progesterone resulted in an increased risk of uterine cancer, because the uterine lining was continually built up by the estrogen and not "shed in a monthly bleed." When estrogen was combined with progesterone, the uterine lining was shed in a monthly bleed due to withdrawal for a few days from progesterone, and there was no increased risk of uterine cancer.

Unfortunately, new information has shown that five years of treatment with both estrogen and progesterone slightly increases the

Estrogen therapy – Where did I put those car keys?

In 2004, the results of the women's Health Initiative Memory study, sponsored by the National Institute of Health (NIH) showed that women taking estrogens might have an increased risk of memory problems. These results seem contrary to what would be expected and haven't been confirmed by other studies.

risk of breast cancer, while treatment with estrogen alone may not. Recent studies have also shown that estrogen-progesterone hormone replacement therapy may increase the risk of heart disease and stroke. Researchers previously thought that hormone replacement therapy was a protection against these diseases.

Because of all the uncertainty about the risk of breast cancer and heart disease with estrogens, many bone specialists use antiresorptive drugs as their first line of treatment for osteoporosis. However, despite the increased risks of breast and uterine cancers, estrogen, in combination with progesterone, and estrogen alone clearly have been shown to reduce fracture rates by about one-third. If your doctor decides that estrogens are right for you, she'll discuss the pros and cons with you and give you the lowest dose available.

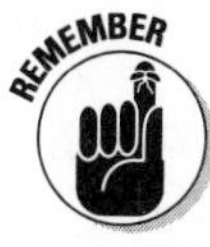

The ideal patient for estrogen therapy in osteoporosis is someone who is in early menopause *and* who is having hot flashes *and* who has had a hysterectomy so that there is no risk of uterine cancer. In this circumstance, estrogen alone in low doses can be used.

Taking estrogen correctly

If your doctor prescribes estrogen, it's available in pills or skin patches. The lowest dose available is 0.3 mg, while the standard dose is 0.625 mg. Estrogen can also be combined with progesterone in hormone replacement therapy (HRT). Some brand names of combination type HRT are Activella, FemHRT, and Prempro.

Estrogen alone or in combination drugs is often taken once a day for most of the month, and then stopped for a few days to allow a withdrawal bleed. Shedding the menstrual lining each month decreases your chance of developing uterine cancer. Your doctor may prescribe a different regimen for taking the drug, so be sure to follow her instructions, because she knows you best.

Whether to use pills or patches is a matter of choice. If you're worried about forgetting a daily pill, patches, which are changed every few days, may be best. Pills may also cause nausea in some people. Pills also need to pass through the liver before being absorbed, whereas patches are directly absorbed into the bloodstream. On the other hand, some people develop skin irritation from the patches and do better with pills.

Pills

Some common brands of estrogen-only pills are

- Cenestin
- Estrace
- Estratab
- Estinyl
- Menest
- Ogen

When taking estrogen pills, you need to remember the following points:

- Take your pill at the same time each day.
- If you miss a pill, don't double the dose the next day.

Combination pills

Your doctor may prescribe combination hormone therapy, which means your pills contain both estrogen and progesterone. This combination means you'll have a withdrawal bleed, similar to a menstrual period, each month. This withdrawal bleed helps protect you from developing uterine cancer. Of course, if you've had your uterus removed (a hysterectomy), there's no reason to take a combination pill.

Combination pills are usually taken for 21 days, and then stopped for one week, during which you'll have a withdrawal bleed.

Some common brand names of combination pills are

- Estratest
- FemHRT
- Prempro

If you're taking a combination pill, you need to remember the following points:

- Take your pill at the same time every day.
- Don't double up the next day if you miss a pill.
- Be aware (and prepared) that you'll have monthly bleed.

Patches

Some common brand names of estrogen patches are

- Alora
- Climara
- Estraderm
- Vivelle
- Vivelle-dot

If you're using estrogen patches, you need to remember the following points:

- Replace your estrogen patches once or twice a week, depending on the brand.
- You can shower or swim with the patch on.
- Rotate the site for your patch every time you change it to avoid skin irritation.
- Most patches need to be placed only on your abdomen or buttocks; don't put them on your breasts or your waist. Don't forget to peel off the backing or they won't stick!

Living with side effects of estrogen

Estrogen can cause some irritating side effects. If you're taking hormone replacement therapy with progesterone, you'll probably have withdrawal bleeding, like a period. This bleeding can be annoying if you thought you were done buying maxi pads ten years ago!

Other side effects of estrogen can include

- Bloating
- Breast tenderness
- Change in sex drive (good or bad!)
- Headaches

- Nausea
- Weight gain

Let your doctor know immediately if you experience

- Abnormal vaginal bleeding
- Breast lumps
- Chest pain or shortness of breath
- Coughing up blood
- Difficulty with your speech
- Pain in your legs, especially your calves
- Severe headache or dizziness
- Weakness or numbness in your arm or leg
- Yellowing of your skin or eyes

Don't take estrogen if you have had blood clots in your veins. (The technical term is *thromboembolic disease.*)

Trying "designer estrogens" (Evista)

Researchers have developed a new class of drugs, called *designer estrogens* that bind only to certain estrogen receptors. (No, these designer estrogens didn't make their debut on a runway.) As a result, these designer estrogens have an effect on bone, but not on the uterus or breast.

One of these medications is known as raloxifene (Evista) and is FDA-approved for the prevention and treatment of postmenopausal osteoporosis. Some evidence has even suggested that raloxifene might lower the risk of breast cancer.

The side effects of raloxifene often limit its use and include the recurrence of hot flashes. You also may have an increased risk of blood clots in the veins, similar to the use of other types of estrogens.

The reason why raloxifene isn't usually considered as the first drug of choice for osteoporosis is that studies haven't shown that the drug protects against fractures, particularly hip fractures, as well as the bisphosphonates.

If you're taking raloxifene, notify your doctor immediately if you notice pain or swelling in your legs, sudden shortness of breath, coughing up blood, or changes in your vision.

On the bright side, raloxifene is also helpful in lowering total and low-density (the "bad" cholesterol) cholesterol levels. Researchers are also testing it to see if it has any effects on heart disease.

Don't take raloxifene if you're

- Pregnant or may become pregnant
- Have a history of blood clots
- Have limited mobility (are in a wheelchair, or in a cast)
- Have liver disease

See the "The Estrogen Replacement Controversy" section earlier in this chapter for more information about taking estrogens.

Calcitonin: An Old Medication Standby

Another drug that inhibits resorption (slowing bone loss) is calcitonin, which was one of the first drugs available to treat osteoporosis. Calcitonin is related to a naturally occurring hormone secreted by a part of the thyroid gland.

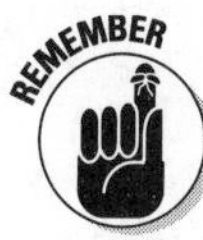

One of the advantages of calcitonin is that it can sometimes alleviate the pain from a skeletal fracture, so physicians often prescribe it to patients who have just experienced a spinal fracture due to osteoporosis. The other major benefit is that it has few side effects. Calcitonin is useful for individuals who can't take bisphosphonates, estrogens, or designer estrogens; unfortunately it's less effective.

Calcitonin is a protein, which means you can't take it in pill form, because your body would digest it before it did you any good. As a result, calcitonin is available in two other forms:

- **Injection:** Available in 50 to 100 IU daily doses
- **Nasal spray:** The most commonly used, you take one daily dose (200 IU)

Injected calcitonin can rarely cause some annoying side effects, such as flushing of your hands and face, nausea, rash, or urinary frequency. The nasal spray form can cause backache, bloody nose or other nasal irritation, and headaches.

Building Bone with Teripeptides

The newest drug on the horizon is the only drug that works by actually stimulating new bone formation. This new molecule is known as *teripeptide,* or human recombinant (meaning that it's manmade in a laboratory) parathyroid hormone (PTH). Bone density in both the spine and hip increase significantly after only 21 months on this medication with the accompanying reduction in fracture rates.

Doctors and researchers have little long-term experience with this hormone, and consequently they don't know of any unusual side effects if the hormone is used for longer periods of time.

The drug does have three major disadvantages:

- It requires one daily injection under the skin.
- It's very expensive.
- Very few insurance companies cover it at this time.

Children or anyone with an elevated calcium level can't take it. Side effects of PTH include dizziness, nausea, and leg cramps.

When to consider prevention

Given the profound effects of corticosteroids, such as prednisone and other prednisonelike drugs, on bone metabolism, you need to take calcium and vitamin D supplements to prevent osteoporosis even if you take prednisone only for a short time. If you take prednisone for a longer period of time, your doctor may order a bone density test ahead of time, assess your risk factors for osteoporosis, and then give you a bisphosphonate as preventive treatment.

Your doctor will adjust the dose of prednisone based upon your risk factors, such as estrogen status, the dose of corticosteroids used, and your baseline bone mineral density as measured by DXA scanning. (See Chapter 9 for more on how DXA scans measure your bone density.)

If you're going to receive an organ transplant, such as liver, kidney, or heart, you're at increased risk for rapid bone loss and your physician may consider preventive therapy in that circumstance as well.

Deciding on testosterone replacement therapy

Testosterone deficiency is a common cause of osteoporosis in men. Low testosterone levels have many causes (see Chapter 4 for more details), but the lower levels are most commonly seen in men who use corticosteroids or those who are undergoing treatment for prostate cancer. So if you're a male with osteoporosis, your doctor might consider testosterone replacement to improve your bone density and prevent fractures.

Testosterone comes in several different forms:

- **Oral:** Oral preparations are difficult, because they cause more liver problems and one needs frequent, high doses.
- **Intramuscular injections:** Injections are inconvenient, but they're less damaging to the liver.
- **Transdermal patches:** Patches also avoid liver toxicity, but they can cause rashes from allergic reactions.
- **Gel:** A new gel applied to the skin called Androgel might be the easiest and safest to use.

Side effects of testosterone include enlargement of the prostate gland, abnormal liver function tests, and abnormal lipid levels. If you're on testosterone replacement, make sure you receive a prostate exam and regular blood tests.

When considering using testosterone, remember these four important points:

- The first line treatment of osteoporosis in men is still a bisphosphonate.

- Testosterone isn't indicated for treatment of osteoporosis in men who have normal testosterone blood levels.

  Don't take testosterone to increase athletic performance.
- If you have the following conditions, don't take testosterone replacement:
  - Breast cancer (men can get breast cancer too)
  - Liver disease

- *Polycythemia* (an illness with a very high amount of red blood cells)
- Prostate cancer

Exploring New Directions in Medication

Researchers and pharmaceutical companies are always developing new medications and figuring out ways to use older medications in new ways. Drugs for osteoporosis are no exception. This section includes some of the "newest kids on the block" in medication options.

Administering bisphosphonates in a new manner

Ten years ago, an intravenous form of bisphosphonate, known as pamidronate, was approved for use in two diseases (Paget's disease, an illness of disordered bone formation, and high calcium levels seen in cancer) . . . but not for osteoporosis.

For osteoporosis, pamidronate (Aredia) is used in a lower dose. Although not FDA-approved, many rheumatologists (including Dr O'Connor) are using pamidronate to treat osteoporosis. This medication is most useful when you have reflux esophagitis (when other bisphosphonate drugs aren't effective because they cause irritation to the esophagus) because pamidronate doesn't cause esophagitis. Therefore many doctors use it in people who can't sit up or who have problems with their esophagus.

Pamidronate is usually given at an infusion center. The dose typically is 30 mg every three to six months. Side effects are uncommon, but include a drop in calcium level or a flulike reaction (consisting of fever and muscle aches). These reactions tend to resolve quickly. It takes about two hours to receive the infusion.

One limitation of the intravenous bisphosphonates is their cost. Because the FDA hasn't approved their use in the treatment of osteoporosis, some insurance companies don't cover the medication.

Another form of intravenous bisphosphonate, which was first studied in 2002 for osteoporosis, is zoledronic acid (Zometa). The drug has been widely used in individuals with bone cancer.

In one study, 351 postmenopausal women received zoledronic acid intravenously once a year. Bone density improved and markers of bone turnover were lowered. In another study, researchers are currently conducting a long-term study in more than 1,700 individuals who have experienced a hip fracture. The question being asked is whether yearly doses of zoledronic acid can prevent future fractures. Keep your eyes open for more results from this study, known as the Horizon future fracture trial.

Combining drug therapies

Using more than one drug to treat difficult cases of osteoporosis is an approach your doctor might try. Although not much evidence supports this approach, your doctor might consider it because doctors frequently use a combination of drugs in treatment of other illnesses, such as high blood pressure or rheumatoid arthritis.

For example, if a man develops osteoporosis on corticosteroid therapy and has a very low testosterone level, he may be prescribed both testosterone replacement and a bisphosphonate.

The effectiveness of a combination therapy isn't clear-cut quite yet. Some evidence in a small population showed that the combination of alendronate and estrogen works better to prevent osteoporosis than taking either drug alone. In contrast to that study, a study with teriparatide and alendronate showed no additional benefit of the combination when compared to each drug used in isolation. These findings are certainly puzzling and warrant repeated investigation.

Using ultra low-dose estrogen

A promising study published in 2004 followed 400 women between the ages of 60 and 80. The women wore an estrogen patch that delivered a very low dose of estrogen. After a two-year period, bone mineral density improved in both the hip and spine. The patients were monitored for endometrial cancer, and none developed. This evidence is promising, but a larger and longer study is needed before anything is conclusive.

Strontium

In 2004, a group of European researchers published the effects of a medication called strontium renelate on vertebral fractures in postmenopausal women. This new medication, taken by mouth, stimulates the formation of new bone as well as decreases bone resorption.

The drug clearly prevented fractures in the spine in a group of high-risk patients. This medication, which has been approved for use in the United Kingdom, but not yet in the United States, is taken once daily and comes in a powder that must be dissolved in water. Patients take the medication at bedtime on an empty stomach.

Side effects include mild nausea and diarrhea, which occur rarely. Don't take this medication if you have a prior history of blood clots.

Tibolone (Livial)

A new type of hormone replacement, called tibolone (Livial), available in Europe and Australia, is a manufactured compound that has properties of several hormones.

It acts like progesterone, *androgen* (a male hormone), and estrogen, and has been referred to as *gonadomimetic* (mimics the function of your ovary). Clearly this medication has the potential to prevent and treat osteoporosis.

A study of 4,000 women is underway to study the benefits and potential side effects of this medication; you can read more about the study and the drug itself at `http://hcp.livial.com`.

One plus to this medication over traditional hormone replacement therapies is that no uterine bleeding occurs in the majority of postmenopausal women taking this drug. If you have a prior history of breast cancer, avoid this drug.

For men with osteoporosis, researchers are developing new designer androgens that might have the desired bony effects, but not the undesirable effects, such as prostate cancer.

Chapter 11

Keeping Bones Strong with Over-the-Counter Supplements

In This Chapter

- Getting enough vitamin D — just how much is the correct amount?
- Overdoing vitamin A — the dangers of taking too much
- Counting on calcium pills to prevent osteoporosis

Specialty stores that tout the latest in vitamin and mineral supplements are flourishing, popping up in shopping centers and malls everywhere. These stores are becoming more and more popular, perhaps due to some surveys that show as many as 53 percent of Americans take a daily vitamin or mineral supplement.

Are you really surprised? Every time you turn on the television or the radio you're constantly bombarded with commercials that encourage you to take certain vitamins, minerals, or other supplements to prevent various diseases and claim that you'll live forever.

Despite all these miracle claims, you may be wondering what exactly are the facts regarding these supplements and your bones? Even though your doctor may not actually write a prescription for them, you still need to carefully consider them just like any other medication that you receive by way of a prescription.

In this chapter, we sort through the information available to help you find a balance between the hype and the facts when taking over-the-counter (OTC) supplements to help with osteoporosis.

Taking enough vitamins . . . or too many?

Although you may take vitamin supplements, do you actually read the contents listed on the bottle to make sure you're getting the exact amount you need? You may figure it's the drug companies' business to figure out all the picky little details, and that you're doing your part to stay healthy by remembering to take what's in the bottle every day.

Unfortunately, vitamin companies work on averages, and what's right for your neighbor may not be right for you. New studies show that some preparations contain vitamins and minerals in amounts that may actually harm you rather than help you, and that others don't contain enough to do any real good.

You need to be proactive and find out what's good — and not good — for you. Become an educated consumer and buy only what you need, and what may be helpful for you.

Why Vitamin D Is a Major Player

Vitamin D's main function is to maintain normal levels of calcium and phosphorus, both vital to the building of healthy bone, in your bloodstream. Vitamin D also assists in bone mineralization. You may hear vitamin D referred to as a hormone as well as a vitamin; this is because vitamin D needs to be converted to an active hormone form to do its job.

If you don't take in enough vitamin D, your bones can become soft and brittle. Children may develop rickets and adults may develop osteomalacia if they don't consume enough vitamin D (see Chapter 4 for more on these diseases).

You can find vitamin D in foods, such as fish and eggs (check out Chapter 5 for more on vitamin D in your diet). Your body also makes vitamin D after your skin is exposed to sunlight. You need sun exposure for 10 to 15 minutes at least two to three times a week to produce the necessary vitamin D. Some people, especially the elderly or homebound, don't get out in the sun this much. Supplementation is most important for these individuals, because they're most likely to be at high risk for fracture.

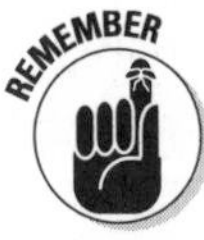

If you live in some areas of the United States where sunlight doesn't provide enough ultraviolet-ray exposure to synthesize vitamin D in the winter months, you may need to consider taking vitamin D supplements. Pollution, cloud cover, and use of sunscreen can also prevent sufficient UV light from reaching the skin to manufacture vitamin D.

You may wonder if a few sessions at the tanning salon would substitute for sunlight in providing ultraviolet light. The answer is: possibly. Tanning salons deliver both ultraviolet A (UVA) and ultraviolet B light (UVB); only UVB synthesizes vitamin D. If you decide to utilize a tanning salon for UV exposure, make sure that the salon is providing UVB rays. Also remember that tanning beds may increase your risk of skin cancer, so talk it over with your doctor before lying down in the bed!

A study done in 2002 showed that 42 percent of African American women were deficient in vitamin D, compared to only 4 percent of Caucasian women. Women of Middle Eastern and Asian descent are also more likely to be vitamin D deficient, partly because darker pigmented skin converts UV rays to vitamin D less efficiently than lighter skin, and partly because women from these cultures may wear clothing that shields them more from the sun's rays.

People older than age 50 are also prone to vitamin D deficiency, because the kidneys are less efficient at converting vitamin D to its active form, and older skin doesn't synthesize vitamin D as well. As a result, your recommended intake of vitamin D becomes higher as you get older (see Table 11-1). In addition, older people are less likely to spend time outdoors, especially in colder climates, where sunlight is already limited. Diseases that interfere with fat absorption can also result in vitamin D deficiency. People with Crohn's disease, cystic fibrosis, celiac disease, and liver disease may need supplementation.

Table 11-1 Recommended Intake of Vitamin D at Different Ages and Stages of Life

Age	*Children*	*Adults*
Birth to 13 years	200 IU/day	
14 to 18 years		200 IU/day
19 to 50 years		200 IU/day
51 to 70 years		400 to 800 IU/day
71 plus years		800 IU/day

Most of the popular multivitamin supplements contain 200 to 400 IU of vitamin D. You need to read the labels carefully to know the amount you're taking.

Checking your vitamin D levels

Your doctor can measure your vitamin D level by blood tests, but the normal values reported by the laboratories are probably too low. Experts now recommend that your blood level of vitamin D needs to be at least 25 nanograms per milliliter (ng/ml). In concert with this amount, in 2005, researchers are also recommending that the upper limit of vitamin D supplementation be increased from 600 IU daily to 800 IU daily in order to maintain a blood level of 25 ng/ml.

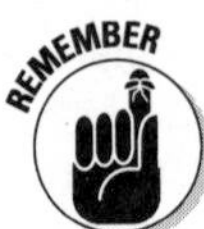

Furthermore, if you're taking alendronate (Fosamax) or risedronate (Actonel) for osteoporosis, then you must have adequate amounts of calcium and vitamin D supplementation in order for the medications to work properly.

Finally, vitamin D deficiency with bone findings showing osteomalacia can look exactly like osteoporosis. Monitoring your vitamin D status if you're undergoing treatment for osteoporosis or if you've had a fracture is critical. Because most patients with vitamin D deficiency and fractures don't have a bone biopsy to look for osteomalacia, the next best step is to restore vitamin D in the blood and observe what happens.

Drugs that interfere with vitamin D absorption

If you're taking certain medications, you may need to supplement vitamin D because the drugs interfere with absorption. Some of the drugs that can interfere with vitamin absorption are

- Anticonvulsants
- Barbiturates
- Cholesterol-lowering medication
- Cortisone
- Digitoxin
- Some laxatives

If you're taking medications that fall into any of these categories, ask your doctor about taking extra vitamin D supplementation.

Correlating vitamin D deficiency and hip fractures

Some evidence suggests that vitamin D deficiency and hip fractures go hand in hand. In fact, one study showed that 50 percent of women hospitalized for hip fractures were vitamin D deficient.

Another long-term study by Harvard Medical School showed that women who supplemented their diet with 500 IU of vitamin D daily reduced their rate of hip fracture by 37 percent, compared to those women whose daily intake of vitamin D was less than 140 IU. This study also showed that 60 percent of women surveyed had intakes of vitamin D that were less than the recommended daily allowance (RDA).

Reducing falls with vitamin D

In 2005, researchers conducted a review of published literature regarding falls in people older than 60 who lived in a community dwelling. The results showed that patients who received various forms of vitamin D supplementation had fewer falls. The investigators conducting this research believe that vitamin D may improve muscle strength, although other factors may also play a part.

Taking in too much vitamin D

You and your doctor may determine that you need to take vitamin D supplements. But can you take in *too* much vitamin D? Absolutely! Because vitamin D is a fat-soluble vitamin, your body stores excess amounts in tissue, instead of washing it out in urine, as water-soluble vitamins are.

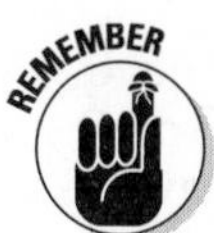

Vitamin D toxicity is almost never caused by excessive sunlight exposure or by dietary intake of vitamin D. The usual cause of vitamin D toxicity is caused by taking in too much vitamin D in the form of supplements.

Some of the symptoms of vitamin D toxicity are

- Constipation
- Decreased appetite or weight loss
- Nausea and vomiting
- Weakness

In addition, too much vitamin D can cause calcium in the blood to rise too high, causing confusion and other changes in mental status. High blood levels of calcium can also cause heart arrhythmias and kidney problems.

Just remember; too much of a good thing, even vitamin D, can be dangerous!

Overdoing Vitamin A

When you think of vitamin supplementation, you probably think in terms of getting enough of a vitamin. The thought of getting too much of a vitamin may not occur to you. However, as is the case with vitamin D, discussed in the previous section, you can take in too much of a vitamin or mineral supplement and end up increasing rather than decreasing your chance of fracture due to osteoporosis.

Vitamin A, which is a fat-soluble vitamin like vitamin D, has come under study recently as a possible culprit in increasing your risk of fracture, not because you may be deficient, but because you may be taking too much vitamin A.

Some studies have shown that supplementing your diet with vitamin A (the retinol form) 10,000 IU daily can increase your chance of bone fracture by up to 40 percent.

Your body still needs some vitamin A to maintain healthy skin, vision, teeth, and hair, among other things. The RDA of vitamin A in adults is between 2,500 IU and 3000 IU per day.

Many vitamin supplements contain up to 10,000 IU of vitamin A, well above the 2,500 RDA. This higher amount may well contribute to bone mineral loss and an increased risk of fracture.

If you take too much vitamin A, not only do you risk the chance of bone fracture, but you also may suffer from vitamin A toxicity. Blood tests may show high levels of liver enzymes if you have vitamin A toxicity, or a higher than normal level of vitamin A. Measurements of the retinol form of vitamin A are commercially available, although not widely ordered. The retinol form of vitamin A, found in liver, egg yolks, cheese, and milk, is the toxic type at high levels, whereas the beta-carotene form, which is contained in carrots, sweet potatoes, spinach, and cantaloupe, seems to be safe.

Signs of vitamin A toxicity include

- Blurred vision
- Decrease in muscle coordination
- Dizziness
- Headache
- Nausea
- Vomiting

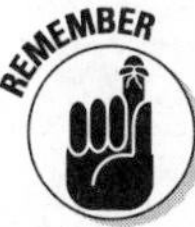

The human body converts beta-carotene, found in many yellow vegetables, to vitamin A, but ingesting beta-carotene doesn't seem to increase risk of fractures, according to several studies. Because of this fact, many multivitamin preparations now include beta-carotene as a substitute for some or all the vitamin A in their preparations. Check your vitamin labels to see if your vitamin A is at least partially being supplied by beta-carotene; if not, look for another supplement.

Confronting the Cacophony of Calcium Supplements

You may drink milk by the gallon and eat cheese by the pound and still wonder if you're getting enough calcium in your diet (see Chapters 5 and 15 for more on calcium in the diet). The best way to get calcium is to take in enough through your diet, but not everyone can do that. For example, for the 25 percent of Americans who are lactose intolerant, incorporating enough calcium into their diet isn't easy (see Chapter 5 for good ideas on getting enough calcium if you're lactose intolerant). Still, 5 percent or more of Americans are worried about getting enough calcium that they take calcium supplements, and many more probably should be worried about their calcium intake.

Recent studies appear to show that calcium alone isn't enough to maintain healthy bones; you also need an adequate amount of vitamin D. (Refer to the section, "Why Vitamin D Is a Major Player" earlier in this chapter for more on the importance of vitamin D in your diet.)

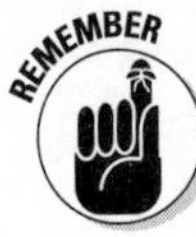

If you're older than 50 years old, you need 1,200 mg of elemental calcium daily to maintain strong bones. More than half of American women may not take in enough calcium without taking supplements. (Check out Chapter 5 for more on getting adequate calcium in your diet.)

Calcium can be confusing, because so many types of calcium supplements are available today. Does your basic drugstore multivitamin contain enough, or do you need to opt for the expensive varieties available only in your local health food store? Do you need to take calcium carbonate, citrate, or one of the other "ates" out there? Is coral calcium all it's cracked up to be?

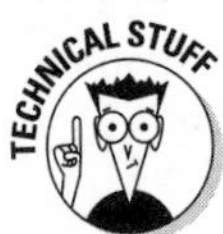

Calcium must be combined with another ingredient, such as citrate or gluconate, to be useful. This is why calcium supplements are manufactured with gluconate or citrate and are listed as, for example, "calcium citrate" rather than just plain calcium.

Reading the labels for elemental calcium

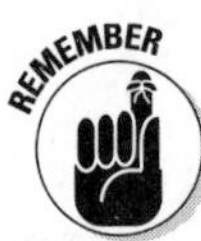

Combining calcium with the different "ates" results in varying amounts of elemental calcium, and elemental calcium is what counts. *Elemental calcium* is the amount of calcium available for absorption into your body. Always check the amount of elemental calcium on the label; this is the only number that counts!

If the amount of elemental calcium isn't listed on the bottle, you can easily figure it out by using these formulas:

- Calcium carbonate contains 40 percent elemental calcium, so 1,000 mg contains 400 mg of elemental calcium.
- Calcium citrate contains 21 percent elemental calcium, so 1,000 mg contains 210 mg of elemental calcium.
- Calcium gluconate contains 9 percent elemental calcium, so 1,000 mg contains 90 mg of elemental calcium.
- Calcium lactate contains 13 percent elemental calcium, so 1,000 mg contains 130 mg of elemental calcium.
- Tribasic calcium phosphate contains 39 percent elemental calcium, so 1,000 mg contains 390 mg of elemental calcium.

Table 11-2 breaks down the amounts of elemental calcium you get when you combine specific amounts of calcium with the added "ate" ingredient.

Table 11-2 Calcium Combinations and the Amount of Elemental Calcium They Contain

Calcium Supplement	*Strength of Tablet in Milligrams*	*Amount of Elemental Calcium Per Tablet in Milligrams*
Calcium carbonate	650	260
	1,250	500
	1,500	600
Calcium citrate	950	200
Calcium gluconate	650	58
	1,000	90
Calcium lactate	650	84
Calcium phosphate, dibasic	500	115
Calcium phosphate, tribasic	800	304

Table 11-2 clearly shows that the best "bang for your buck" in calcium comes from calcium carbonate supplements; they contain 40 percent elemental calcium. The good news is that calcium carbonate is also the cheapest and most common source of calcium in supplements. The downside of calcium carbonate is that it can cause gas, constipation, reflux, and bloating.

Ingesting your daily calcium

You need to remember these few caveats when you take your daily calcium:

- **If you're taking a large amount, such as 1,000 mg, don't take it all at once.** Your body can absorb only 500 mg of calcium at one time. Split your doses up into morning and evening, if you can remember to take two pills each day!

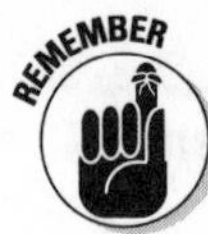

- **Take your calcium carbonate with meals.** It requires additional acid to digest.

  However, calcium citrate, which is the best-absorbed form of calcium supplement, is maximally absorbed if taken an hour or so after meals. Calcium citrate also comes in a liquid form that may be less irritating to intestinal walls. If you're taking any type of acid blockers, your body will better absorb calcium citrate than other types of calcium.
- **If your meal contained a large amount of fiber, wait one to two hours before taking your calcium or it may not be well absorbed.** Fiber can move stomach contents through your intestines too fast for calcium to be well absorbed.
- **Drink a full glass of water or juice when you take your pill.** Doing so helps speed absorption and also helps you "wash the pill down" without getting it stuck in your throat, if you have difficulty swallowing pills.
- **If you're on other medications, don't ingest your calcium pill within one to two hours of your other medications.** Doing so can interfere with absorption of some medications; discuss timing of multiple medications with your doctor.

Does it sound like you'll need a calendar to keep all this information straight? You're probably right! Just make sure you plan out when to take all your meds and supplements and then stick to that schedule. You can also consider taking a combination supplement (check out "Combining calcium and other vitamins and minerals" later in this chapter.)

Calcium interactions

A large number of medications and foods can interact with calcium. Be aware of the following possible interactions:

- **Caffeine:** High caffeine intake can cause excess urinary excretion.
- **Dilantin:** Don't take it within one to three hours of calcium, or the effects of both medications can be decreased.
- **Iron:** Don't take iron and calcium at the same time, because each can interfere with the other's absorption.
- **Laxatives:** Anything that moves substances through the intestine very quickly can result in calcium being excreted before it's absorbed.

- **Oxalic acid:** You find this acid in spinach, soybeans, and coca; it absorbs calcium found in these substances. It doesn't affect calcium taken in from other sources at the same time.
- **Excess phosphorus and magnesium:** The absorption of phosphorus and magnesium requires vitamin D. If you consume these minerals in excess amounts, they'll use up more vitamin D, leaving less available for calcium absorption.
- **Tannins in tea:** They may interfere with calcium absorption.
- **Tetracycline:** Calcium supplements taken at the same time may decrease the efficacy of this antibiotic; separate doses of calcium and tetracycline by one to three hours.
- **Thyroid medication:** Calcium supplements can interfere with effectiveness of thyroid medication. Take them at least two to three hours apart.

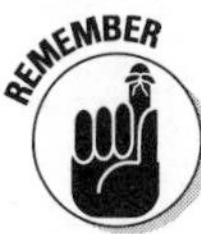

Count calcium from fortified sources such as milk or juice as a supplement. Don't take fortified foods with drugs that shouldn't be taken with supplements!

Making sure your calcium dissolves

Swallowing a calcium pill is one thing; making sure that the pill dissolves quickly enough to be properly absorbed is something different.

A quick test to see if your supplement is sufficiently dissolvable is to drop one into a glass of warm water or vinegar and see if it dissolves within a half-hour. If it does, it's sufficiently dissolvable. You don't want it to have any chunks left at the bottom of the glass.

The coral calcium controversy

Coral calcium is most often sold in health food stores, at prices far above your average calcium pill. Coral calcium is simply calcium carbonate, plus small amounts of magnesium with lead.

Some individuals have made claims that coral calcium cures everything from osteoporosis to cancer, but these claims have been debunked. No proof shows that coral calcium works any better than any other calcium carbonate. Save yourself a few bucks and skip the coral calcium.

Another way to be sure your pill will be absorbed is to buy only supplements with "USP" (which stands for US Pharmacoeia) on them. Pills with the label are guaranteed to meet the standard set for adequate absorption.

Of course, if you take chewable or liquid supplements, you don't have to worry about whether or not they're going to dissolve properly; at least you won't as long as you chew thoroughly before swallowing.

Table 11-3 lists the most commonly used calcium supplements.

Table 11-3 The Most Common Calcium Supplements

Calcium Supplement	*Type of Calcium*	*Amount of Elemental Calcium*
Caltrate 600 mg	Calcium carbonate	600 mg
Citracel 950 mg	Calcium citrate	200 mg
Os-Cal 500	Calcium carbonate	500 mg
TUMS regular	Calcium carbonate	200 mg
TUMS ultra	Calcium carbonate	400 mg
Viactiv	Calcium carbonate	500 mg

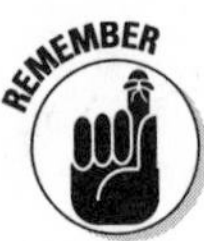

Always check to see how much vitamin D is included with your calcium supplements.

Getting the lead out

You may want to increase your calcium levels, but are concerned that doing so will also increase the amount of lead you ingest, possibly leaving you at risk for lead poisoning. The truth is, many calcium compounds do contain small amounts of lead, because lead and calcium are found together in marine calcareous deposits.

The Food and Drug Administration (FDA) has set an upper limit on acceptable amounts of lead in 1,000 milligrams of calcium as 7.5 micrograms, but this amount greatly exceeds the 6 micrograms per day experts recommend as safe for total lead ingestion.

Supplements with measurable lead contained no more than 1 to 2 micrograms, but the combination of overusing of calcium and ingesting foods high in lead could cause an amount exceeding the daily limit. Many companies have reduced lead content in supplements by refining it out or by using calcium deposits with lower lead content. Nearly 70 percent of supplements now have amounts of lead below detection levels.

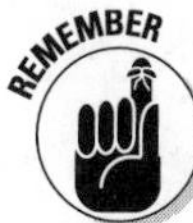

Fortunately, calcium blocks the absorption of lead in your intestine, because both are absorbed at the same site, and the site prefers calcium. So lead ingested along with calcium may be less harmful than lead ingested from other substances.

Looking for supplements that state they test for lead content is worthwhile, but don't focus so much on the dangers of lead that you stop taking any calcium supplements at all. Even more important, don't overdose by taking more pills than you need.

Unacceptable levels of lead, in addition to other heavy metals, such as arsenic, have also been found in another calcium source sold in some health food stores, bone meal. Bone meal is made from processed crushed cattle or horse bone. Avoid using bone meal as a calcium supplement!

Combining calcium and other vitamins and minerals

Some manufacturers have combined calcium with other necessary elements in one supplement. If you're the type of person who wants to take just one pill and forget about the rest, or if you have a tendency to forget half your pills on a daily basis, taking one of these pills may appeal to you.

Combining calcium and vitamin D

Some supplements contain both calcium and vitamin D, which is necessary for calcium absorption. Taking one of these supplements is one way of assuring that you're getting enough of both, but be especially careful not to take more than the recommended dose. You don't want to overdose on them both.

Getting your calcium from multivitamins

You may wonder why you can't just swallow your multivitamin and forget about all these other complicated supplements. You could, if you can find a multivitamin that contained an adequate amount of calcium. However, most multivitamins contain only 200 mg, not enough to supply your daily requirement.

Creating a dream team: Calcium and chocolate!

A new supplement on the market called Viactiv puts the almost unbeatable combination of chewable chocolate and calcium together. These bite-sized chews also contain vitamins D and K along with calcium carbonate. Although the label says the calcium amount is 500 mg, remember that only 40 percent, or 200 mg, of calcium carbonate is absorbable.

Another downside of this seemingly unbeatable combination is that it does contain some sugar, and therefore a small amount of calories. And you do have the possibility of becoming hooked on these little candies and being tempted to overindulge. Take only if you have adequate willpower to resist emptying the box!

Because this supplement has Vitamin K in it, you can't take it if you take Coumadin (a blood thinner).

Antacids for your bones?

What do you already have in your medicine cabinet that can boost your calcium intake? Antacid tablets. But wait — before you throw out your calcium supplements from the health food store, you may want to consider whether antacids are really the best source of calcium supplementation. Consider the following:

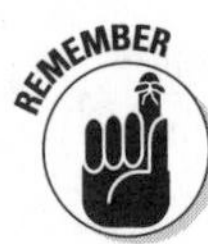

- Antacids contain the cheapest and best-absorbed form of calcium, calcium carbonate. Some antacids also contain aluminum, which actually interferes with calcium absorption by binding with phosphorus in the intestines.
- Don't use antacids containing aluminum as a source of calcium supplementation!
- Calcium requires an acidic environment to be well absorbed. Antacids, by definition, decrease stomach acid, and so may result in less calcium being absorbed than a calcium supplement without acid reducers.
- Some antacids have no active ingredients other than calcium carbonate, which also acts as an acid reducer. These antacid tablets are often chewable, easy to take, reasonably priced, and can be the best way to get your daily dose of calcium. Just be careful to check and see how much calcium is in your antacid to be sure that you're taking enough!

Taking calcium when you have other medical conditions

Some medical conditions can affect your use of calcium supplements. First, talk to your doctor and pharmacist and exercise extreme caution if you have any condition known to elevate the amount of calcium in your blood.

Three important conditions to consider are

- **Hyperparathyroidism:** With this condition your parathyroid gland makes too much parathyroid hormone. This hormone increases calcium absorption, and hence, extra calcium supplementation can lead to dangerously high blood calcium levels. High blood calcium levels can cause confusion, muscle weakness, and abnormal heart rhythms, to list just a few of the problems.
- **Kidney stones:** Occasionally patients with certain types of kidney stones tend to have elevated calcium levels in their urine. Discuss calcium supplementation with your physician if you have a history of kidney stones or any other problem with your kidneys.
- **Sarcoidosis:** This is a benign illness of unknown cause characterized by granuloma formation in many organs. About one quarter of individuals have elevated blood calcium levels. Therefore if you have sarcoidosis, you must discuss the safety of calcium and vitamin D supplementation with your physician.

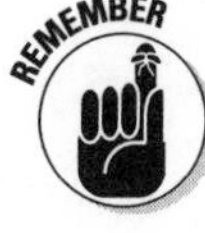

If you're diagnosed with one of these conditions, make sure that you alert your doctor and pharmacist about any OTC supplements that you take. Remember that the OTC supplements are drugs, and your physician needs to monitor them just like prescription meds!

Chapter 12

Managing Pain from Osteoporosis

In This Chapter

- Dealing with the pain of osteoporosis
- Finding medication that works for you
- Being aware of possible side effects
- Handling pain without medication

Osteoporosis isn't painful until you've fractured something. This important fact often confuses people. You can have a significant reduction in bone density and have no symptoms at all.

If you're one of the unlucky people who developed a fracture from osteoporosis, you already know about the pain from the broken bone. For instance, a broken hip or wrist can cause immediate pain and inability to use the hip or wrist. Osteoporosis also can cause rib fractures from minimal trauma. These typically cause severe pain in various areas of the rib cage. (See Chapter 7 for more on how your "bones go bad" without your realizing it until you break something.)

In contrast, if you've fractured a bone in your spine, you may still be able to function normally, although you may notice that you're getting shorter progressively. And you may have pain in your back that you simply dismiss as "getting older." Most people who fracture a vertebra due to osteoporosis don't have sudden onset of severe back pain. Only about one-third of patients with osteoporotic-related spinal fractures actually come to medical attention because of pain. Unfortunately, for those who do experience pain from spinal fracture, the pain can be severe and unrelenting.

To keep the pain from any type of fracture to a minimum, you may need to utilize several different pain-relieving techniques. Working with your doctor to find the right combination of drug therapy, exercise, or manipulation is the best approach to take.

Decreasing your pain can help keep you on your feet, and staying mobile helps keep your bones strong. In this chapter, we discuss ways you can deal with the pain resulting from a fracture so your osteoporosis doesn't drastically alter your life.

Recognizing the Real Pain of Osteoporosis

Pain not only hurts, but it also has long-lasting consequences beyond the immediate discomfort. Acute pain, which occurs suddenly after an injury, is sometimes more bearable than chronic pain because you know acute pain will go away — usually sooner rather than later! Chronic pain, which lasts more than three months, can alter your lifestyle as well as your physical and mental states.

Everyone has a different tolerance to pain. In some individuals, chronic pain can make them angry, depressed, and even frustrated. It can take the joy out of daily events, and leave you with a fear of doing anything that might cause more pain.

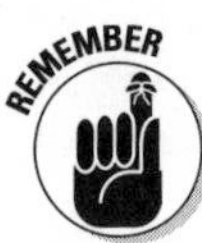

Because osteoporosis is a chronic condition, you may be dealing with both acute and chronic pain. Pain from rib fractures and spinal fractures often lasts for three months or longer. The pain from hip fractures and from wrist fractures is often shorter, because the hip fracture can be surgically repaired and the wrist fracture can be casted. The pain of osteoporosis doesn't come just from fractures; damage to muscles from abnormal posture caused by vertebral compression fractures or from muscles tightening in reaction to discomfort can also cause chronic pain.

If you fall and break a bone, you'll obviously feel the immediate pain; however, vertebral compression fractures usually occur without any sort of trauma. In fact, 30 percent occur while you're in bed (no, not from doing *that!*)!

Because a fractured vertebra may not be as obvious to others or to yourself as that of a visible break, such as a deformity from wrist fracture, you may not realize at first that your pain is from osteoporosis. After you recognize the pain for what it is, several options are available to help you alleviate the pain of osteoporosis.

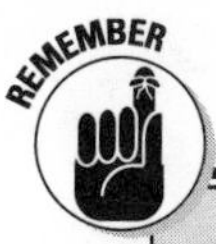

What's hurting today?

Many of you may wake up each morning and do a mental inventory, sort of a "What's hurting today?" laundry list. Taking this step is actually a good idea, as long as you don't make it the highlight of your day!

Being aware of what's normal for you may help you be more aware when something has changed for the worse; the sooner you get treatment, the sooner you'll start to feel better.

Making notes of any new pain that shows up is a good idea. You can jot down the type of pain (sharp, dull, stabbing, deep), the location, and exactly when it started to hurt. You also need to keep track of what makes the pain hurt worse, and what makes it feel better.

Your doctor will love you if you can answer questions like, "When did the pain start?" by simply referring to your notes rather than vaguely guessing the answers. In fact, keeping track — without being obsessive about it — is a good idea with all health problems, not just those related to osteoporosis.

"Oh, My Aching Back!"

Does your back hurt? If so, you're in good company. Nearly 45 percent of Americans complain of aching backs. Although you may think your aching back is caused by osteoporosis, only about half the people who are diagnosed with spinal fractures complain of pain.

As you know by now from reading this chapter, back pain can be caused by vertebral compression fractures; yet you still need to check with your doctor about other potential causes as well. And because 25 percent of all postmenopausal women will experience a vertebral compression fracture, osteoporosis still accounts for a lot of aching backs! Vertebral compression fractures account for around 50 percent of all osteoporotic fractures, and one-third of women older than age 65 have at least one in their lifetime.

Because back pain is so common, many people never follow up with their doctor about it, dismissing it as just another part of aging. This could be part of the reason that two-thirds of spinal fractures are never diagnosed. Because of this statistic, anyone older than 55 who has sudden onset of back pain needs to be evaluated for osteoporosis.

Treating Acute Pain from a Fracture

If you have a fracture other than a vertebral fracture, you feel *acute,* or sudden pain, and often some deformity that's clearly visible. Often, you won't be able to move the broken bone.

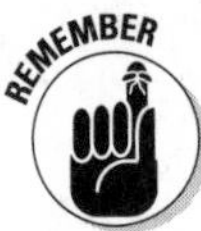

Because a fracture causes immediate pain and disability, you need to see a doctor immediately. Until you get to a doctor, immobilize the broken bone with a splint or sling, if you break an arm or wrist. If you think your hip is broken, don't try to walk on it. If you have to go upstairs to get to a phone, try not to put any stress on the broken side.

After the doctor has worked to fix your fracture, discuss pain medications and treatments with him. A complete description of all pain-relieving medications is far beyond the scope of this book. Nonetheless, the next section briefly mentions some of the medications that doctors often prescribe for a short time after a painful fractured bone.

Narcotic medications for short-term pain

Initial pain from a broken bone can be treated with narcotic painkillers, provided you aren't susceptible to their side effects. Narcotics may cause disorientation, dizziness, respiratory depression, and constipation, so if your doctor thinks any of those side effects may be a big problem for you, he may want you to take them for as short a time as possible.

We list some of the most common narcotic pain medications in Table 12-1.

Table 12-1 Some Common Pain Relievers

Familiar Name	*Actual Composition*
Tylenol #3	Acetaminophen 300 mg + codeine 30 mg
Percocet 7.5	Acetaminophen 325 mg + oxycodone 7.5 mg
Percodan	Aspirin 325 mg + oxycodone 7.5

Familiar Name	Actual Composition
Vicodan	Acetaminophen 500 mg + hydrocodone bitartrate 5 mg
Duragesic patch	Pure narcotic (fentanyl) (varying doses in long-acting patch format)
Oxycontin IR	Pure narcotic (oxycodone) (comes in varying doses)

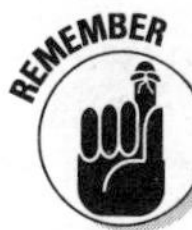

One important thing to look at with any prescribed or over-the-counter (OTC) medication is whether the drug contains more than one type of medicine. For example, if your doctor prescribes Tylenol #3 for you, she's really prescribing 300 mg of acetaminophen with 30 mg of codeine. This information is important if you're also taking acetaminophen separately because you increase the chance of overdose and/or drug interactions if you don't know exactly what's in the combination pill you're taking.

When taking narcotic medications to treat short-term pain, remember these do's and don'ts:

Do:

- Take your medicine the way the doctor prescribed. Never "double up" on your dose without discussing it with her.
- Be especially careful when moving around. Many narcotics make you drowsy and you don't need another fall!
- Take only what you need to control the pain; narcotics can be addicting.
- Tell your doctor if you have a rash, shortness of breath, or any other unusual reaction to your medication.
- Take a stool softener if you're prone to constipation.

Don't:

- Avoid taking medication if you need it.
- Take a friend's medication because "she had the same thing and this worked for her."

OTC analgesics or NSAIDs?

A quick trip to the drugstore to look for pain medications when you're hurting can leave you in more pain from brain strain. So many little bottles of pills, and all claiming to be the best, or at least "just as good" as the others. How do you know what works best when you have pain?

We strongly recommend that if you have serious pain from a fracture, that you consult your physician for proper instructions in pain relief medications. Many OTC *analgesics* (pain relievers) can cause drug-to-drug interactions or some other toxicity. (Any medication that relieves pain is referred to as an analgesic regardless of how it works.)

That being said, you'll find that OTC pain medicines fall into two categories: acetaminophen and nonsteroidal anti-inflammatory medications (NSAIDs).

Asking for acetaminophen

You're not likely to walk into the drugstore and ask for acetaminophen — even if you can pronounce it! Acetaminophen is better known as Tylenol.

Acetaminophen has some benefits over NSAIDs and also some disadvantages. On the plus side:

- Acetaminophen is easier on your stomach.
- It generally causes less irritation.

On the negative side:

- Acetaminophen doesn't reduce inflammation.
- Taking more than the recommended dosage of acetaminophen, 4,000 mg per day, can lead to liver failure. The risk for liver failure is especially high if you mix acetaminophen with alcohol.
- Acetaminophen can also cause blood thinning.

Turning to NSAIDs

If your doctor recommends an NSAID for pain relief, you can spend hours picking up drug store bottles and comparing television commercials. They all claim so many benefits; should you go with "what doctors recommend most" or "the one hospitals use"?

NSAID is short for nonsteroidal anti-inflammatory drug, which may not seem any clearer to you at first. If you break it down word by word, however, you get a pretty good definition of what an NSAID is. It's "not a steroid," so it doesn't have the bone-damaging characteristics that steroids do (see Chapter 3 for more on the risks of corticosteroids on your bones). However an NSAID is an anti-inflammatory (against *inflammation,* or the warmth and swelling you can have from an irritated or infected body part). NSAIDs inhibit an enzyme called *cyclooxygenase* (COX for short). (See the sidebar "What's COX got to do with it?" in this chapter, for more information on how NSAIDs work.)

NSAIDs are further divided into three different types. We list each type with an example:

- **COX-1 type:** naproxen (Aleve), ibuprofen (Advil and Motrin)
- **COX-2 type:** celecoxib (Celebrex) — prescription only
- **Salicylates:** aspirin

As for which NSAID is best for you, ask your doctor first. Many NSAIDs are available over the counter, such as aspirin, ibuprofen, and naproxen. Some are available by prescription only.

Remember that NSAIDs all have similar side effects, which can be harmful if you take more than the prescribed dose. For example, if your doctor gives you a prescription for extra-strength ibuprofen, don't buy another NSAID over the counter, such as Aleve, aspirin, or Advil, and take that as well. The resulting NSAID overdose can be dangerous, causing stomach irritation or bleeding.

What's COX got to do with it?

The first NSAID ever developed was aspirin. It relieves pain by inhibiting cyclooxygenase (COX) enzymes. When these enzymes are inhibited, there is a reduction in swelling. Undoubtedly you've heard a lot about these enzymes because of the drug Vioxx. (The Food and Drug Administration took it off the market in 2004 after some research showed that it might lead to heart attacks and heart damage.) More than 30 different kinds of NSAIDs are available, and they're all related to aspirin in the sense that they all inhibit COX enzymes. They differ in their dosing and side effects. Many are available over the counter. (See "Non-narcotic prescription pain medications" in this chapter for more info.)

Important things to know about NSAIDs:

- You can't take Advil, Motrin, or ibuprofen (all the same thing!) if you have a predisposition to gastroesophageal reflux, stomach ulcers, renal disease, liver disease, or congestive heart failure.

- If you're taking warfarin (Coumadin), you need to be especially careful about taking any other medications, particularly NSAIDs. (Even acetaminophen can interact with Coumadin, a blood thinner.) NSAIDs can increase bleeding, and the combination can lead to a serious gastrointestinal (GI) bleed.

  In the general population, the risk of GI bleeding associated with NSAIDs use is about 1 percent, but the risk rises to 3 to 4 percent in those ages 60 and older.

  You have a higher risk of GI bleeding if you:

  - Are 65 or older
  - Have a history of stomach ulcers
  - Are taking corticosteroids
  - Are taking Coumadin
  - Are taking more than one NSAID

- Taking single drugs, such as plain aspirin, can be better than taking combination drugs, such as Excedrin, which contains acetaminophen as well as aspirin and also a hefty dose of caffeine. Combination drugs may give you ingredients you don't need and also increase the chance of drug interactions.

Non-narcotic prescription pain medications

At this book's writing, the FDA is reviewing the safety and benefits of taking NSAIDs called COX-2 inhibitors. (See the sidebar "What's COX got to do with it?" in this chapter, for more info.) These COX 2 inhibitors NSAIDs include Vioxx, Bextra, and Celebrex, which are all prescription medications. An expert panel recently testified for the FDA and recommended that Celebrex stay on the market. (Vioxx was taken off the market in mid-2004, Bextra in 2005.)

Don't continue to take these medications without discussing them with your doctor and reviewing together the new information about possible heart attacks while taking these drugs. A good place to read about this complex and controversial topic is the

American College of Rheumatology Web site (www.rheumatology.org/publications/hotline/0305NSAIDs.asp).

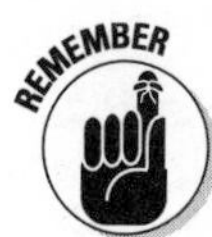

One medication often neglected in the treatment of pain due to fractures is calcitonin. (We discuss calcitonin in Chapter 10.) This hormone nasal spray is used to build bone density, but it also can relieve pain. (Calcitonin is also available in a subcutaneous injection.) Dr. O'Connor often uses this drug in hospitalized patients with pain from a new spinal fracture due to osteoporosis.

Your doctor may also prescribe medications such as antidepressants (amitriptylene). You may protest that you're not depressed; you're in pain! But if your doctor suggests them, give them a try. They modify the way your nervous system processes pain and how the brain processes the signals from the nervous system. Another drug that affects the way the brain processes pain is gabapentin (Neurontin), an antiseizure medication. We discuss Neurontin in the section "Seeing a pain management guru," later in this chapter.

Another medication used to block pain may be familiar if you think back to your last dentist visit to have a cavity filled. Prior to the drilling, you probably received an injection of novocaine (or lidocaine). This numbing medication is now available in patch form that you can apply to your skin. It may be beneficial for relief of back pain, and your doctor may prescribe it for the pain you're experiencing from an osteoporotic fracture. The patch of lidocaine is called Lidoderm; you leave the patch on for 12 hours and then remove it. Twelve hours later, you reapply another patch.

Treating Chronic Pain: What to Do When Pain Goes On and On

If you break a bone, you expect a certain amount of pain. But what do you do when the end of the painful experience never seems to end? If you have a fracture, healing should occur within a few months. If you're still having pain after three months, ask your doctor why.

When pain medication makes you woozy

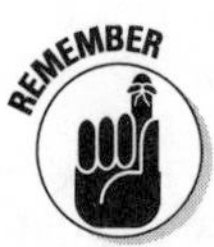

Whenever you start a new medication, such as certain pain relievers with narcotics or even an OTC medicine, you have some potential for dizziness and wooziness, especially when you first get up and stand after sitting for a long time. Be particularly careful because one of the main risks for osteoporotic fracture is falling (see Chapter 13 for more on how to prevent falls).

In fact, older people have a 10 to 25 percent higher risk of having adverse reactions to drugs, so be vigilant about using handrails or bracing yourself when you stand up. Many older people don't metabolize medicine as quickly as they used to, so the effects may last longer. Less medication may be needed as well, because many people older than 65 need a lower dose of medication to get good relief. Start out with a low dose and increase if needed to decrease the chance of dizziness or confusion from your medicine. See the section "Narcotic medications for short-term pain," earlier in this chapter for more suggestions on taking narcotics safely.

Taking more than one medication

Opening your medicine cabinet may be a little like Pandora's box; all sorts of things may come out, and some of them may not be good for you.

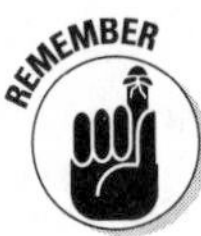

The most important thing to look for when taking more than one medication is the way your medications react with each other. Read the labels and make sure you're not taking the same medication twice, under different name brands. Doing so is particularly important if you're taking a medication that can cause stomach irritation and possible bleeding, such as aspirin or ibuprofen.

Always tell your doctor about all your medications and their doses, even if they're OTC, including all supplements, herbs, and drugs from a health food store. And if you have "leftover" pain medicines from a previous illness, make sure you check the expiration date before taking them, because drugs can lose their potency after they expire. Be sure to check with your doctor to make sure using them is okay.

Studies have shown that people older than 65 take three times as many prescription medications as the general population. People older than 65 also are most likely to take their medicines incorrectly. If your doctor prescribes pain medication for chronic pain, you need to be very careful to take it correctly and to keep track of any side effects.

Keeping an eye on addiction

Becoming dependent on pain medication is possible, but don't be overly concerned if you have chronic pain. Most studies show that more people older than 65 are undermedicated for chronic pain rather than overmedicated. Addiction can also occur if you develop a tolerance to the beneficial effect of a narcotic. Are you scratching your head and wondering what that means? It means that the amount of drug that works to decrease your pain is no longer enough, and you need to gradually increase the dose in order to achieve the same pain relief.

That being said, some people do become dependent on narcotics, even when they start out taking them for a legitimate reason. To avoid problems with dependency, take pain medication only when you really need it, not just because "it's been four hours."

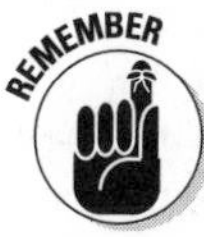

The exception is when your doctor specifically tells you to take your medication on a schedule so your pain doesn't become severe. Studies show that people who need pain medication because they're in pain are able to stop the medication without difficulty when they no longer have pain. Don't be afraid to use your pain medication in the way it's intended.

Dealing with Pain without Medication

Although popping a pill may be easy for instant relief, you (and your doctor) need to aim pain treatment at more than temporary relief. The nonmedication methods in this section may relieve pain and keep it from coming *back*.

Heating it up or cooling it down

Heat packs and/or ice packs can be very helpful for relieving pain, especially if the pain is localized to one spot. If you're very stiff in the morning, standing in the warm shower can be enough to loosen you up, but be sure you're using your handrails! Cold packs can be wonderful for reducing swelling and inflammation, and can reduce pain by temporarily numbing the nerves.

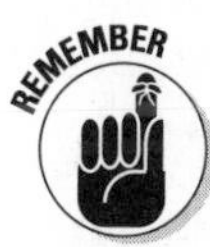

You don't have to buy expensive heat and ice packs, although you can use the electric heating pads to cover larger areas, and some are especially designed for your neck or back. Some apply moist heat. However, if you want to make your own hot packs, you can warm slightly dampened towels in the microwave. Remember that microwaves don't apply heat evenly, and make sure the towel doesn't get too hot in one spot; you could end up with a painful burn in addition to your other aches and pains.

Frozen vegetables, especially peas, which can be made to conform to oddly shaped areas, make very good cold packs. Of course, you need to use the vegetables in the bag, not the ones in a box! Crushed ice in a resealable baggie also makes a good ice pack.

Using physical therapy

Physical therapy can help you maintain and improve the muscle strength you have, as well as increase your energy levels and raise your levels of *endorphins* (natural painkillers released by your body).

Some physical therapists come directly to your home and can help you assess your home for possible sources of injury. A physical therapist can assess your gait, help you improve your posture, reduce muscle strain, and help strengthen weakened or problem areas with specific exercises. (Refer to Chapter 13 for more on what a physical therapist does.)

Many insurance plans cover part or all the cost of physical therapy, which can become quite costly if you go two to three times a week. (See Chapter 8 for more on insurance coverage.) Your plan may only cover if you go to a certain therapist, so make sure you check with the physical therapist's office to see if it's part of your plan.

Exercising to get rid of pain

When you're hurting, the last thing you may want to do is exercise, but exercise keeps you limber, builds your strength, and increases your energy level. The key to exercise is finding the right kind, not overdoing when you first begin, and not giving it up after a short time. (See Chapter 6 for more on exercising if you have osteoporosis.)

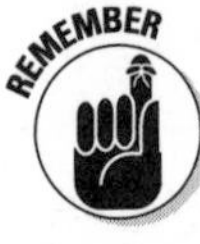

Aquatic physical therapy is one of Dr. O'Connor's favorite prescriptions after the acute injury has started to heal. Walking in a pool filled with very warm water is beneficial in relieving pain and in beginning the muscle-strengthening process. Swimming, although not a weight-bearing exercise and therefore not helpful to improve bone mass, is a good exercise for weakened or damaged tissue. Warm water may also be wonderful for relieving muscle spasm.

Some insurance companies also cover part of the cost of pool or gym membership, realizing that exercise helps reduce health problems overall. You may have to pay upfront and be reimbursed; check with your insurance company for what it requires.

Exploring TENS units

A Transcutaneous Electrical Nerve Stimulation (TENS) unit uses electrical impulses to block pain signals. A technician places electrodes on your skin near the site that is hurting, and transmits a mild electrical current through them, blocking the sensation of pain for several hours.

TENS units cost around $100, and the electrodes run around $30 for a pack of four. Electrodes are good for between 15 to 30 uses. TENS units run on batteries, and most are small enough to hook to your belt so you can keep moving while you're wearing one.

Use a TENS unit only under the supervision of your doctor or physical therapist; your insurance may reimburse the cost as long as you have a prescription for the unit. You can also rent a TENS unit before buying one to make sure it's going to help you with your pain. Many medical companies let you rent one for a month and apply the rental fee to the purchase price if you decide to buy the unit.

If you have a pacemaker, you may not be able to use a TENS unit without interfering with your pacemaker. Talk to your doctor before considering a TENS unit.

Trying acupuncture for chronic pain

The word "acupuncture" may have you envisioning small dark rooms with ancient Chinese chanting in the background. However, in the last few years, acupuncture has become a more widely used and accepted method for dealing with chronic pain.

An acupuncturist inserts very thin needles, about the width of a strand of hair, into certain points of your body to stimulate nerve endings and release endorphins. You may need six or more treatments before you have significant pain relief.

Acupuncture became an officially recognized treatment for pain by the National Institutes of Health (NIH) in 1997. Physicians can be certified in acupuncture after taking a 200-to-300-hour training course. They're then members of the American Academy of Medical Acupuncture (AAMA). Chiropractors and *naturopaths* (practitioners that treat health problems by using noninvasive natural medicine) can also be certified in acupuncture by completing a 200-to-300-hour course, and can then be approved by their state licensing boards to provide acupuncture. The National Certification Commission can also certify acupuncturists for Acupuncture and Oriental Medicine (NCCAOM).

A variation of acupuncture is *acupressure,* where pressure is applied to certain "trigger points" to relieve pain. An instructor may be able to show you this technique so that you can do it at home.

Massaging away the pain

You can also use massage therapy to decrease pain, relax muscles, and relieve tension. Some malls have massage therapists set up so you can shop and then drop onto the table for some relaxation, but make sure the person doing your massage is a trained therapist.

Massage therapists should be graduates of an institution accredited by the Commission for Massage Training Accreditation (COMTA) and should also be members of the American Massage Therapy Association (AMTA).

If you have osteoporosis, don't allow a therapist to deep massage near your spine. The pressure can cause fractures.

Bracing yourself, internally and externally

Spinal fractures are less likely to cause pain and deformity if they're braced; that is, if the broken bones are held in place to keep your spine in the best possible alignment. Bones can be held in place externally, by the wearing of a back brace, or internally, by a newer technique called *percutaneous vertebroplasty.*

External braces are often worn only during the acute phase after injury, because long-term use may weaken your back muscles. Meanwhile, percutaneous vertebroplasty involves stabilizing the fracture by injecting an acrylic cement into the broken areas of the vertebrae. An even newer technique called *kyphoplasty* inserts acrylic cement after inserting a balloon device into the vertebrae to try and restore the vertebrae to their normal position. This procedure reduces the deformity known as a *dowager's hump* that develops when the vertebrae collapse. See Chapter 13 for more on both procedures.

Coping with pain psychologically

Your mind is a powerful thing. In fact, "mind over matter" actually can reduce pain. Several different techniques use your mind to overcome pain:

- **Biofeedback:** With this technique, you discover how to use your body's response to decrease pain and stress through positive reinforcement. Often the technique is first taught with the use of a machine that records your heart rate and other vital signs as they change in response to stimuli.

  Eventually you figure out how to respond positively to pain by relaxing muscles, breathing deeply, or by using visual imagery to distract you from the pain.
- **Guided imagery:** This technique induces relaxation and decreases tension and anxiety by using visual images.
- **Hypnosis:** This technique puts you into a "trance state" characterized by extreme suggestibility and relaxation. A therapist may demonstrate a type of self-hypnosis similar to relaxation training so you can use it at home yourself.
- **Relaxation training:** This technique shows you how to relax tense muscles and reduce anxiety that can intensify pain.
- **Music therapy:** You can use this technique in conjunction with relaxation therapy to decrease anxiety and relax tense muscles.

You can also incorporate several of these methods together, such as relaxation training, music therapy, and biofeedback, to help cope with pain.

Seeing a pain management guru

You also have the option of seeing a pain management specialist. Typically a pain management specialist is an anesthesiologist with special interest in pain who is trained to give nerve blocks and other special procedures.

Pain management specialists often use a medication referred to as gabapentin (Neurontin) for pain. Originally the FDA approved this drug for treatment of seizures, but physicians discovered that it was useful for the pain that occurs after shingles and for the pain that occurs from damaged peripheral nerves, as seen in diabetes. Now doctors use gabapentin as a medication for treatment of all kinds of pain, as well as a number of other diseases.

Some pain management physicians are anesthesiologists with special training in performing nerve blocks as well as other sophisticated procedures designed to inhibit the impulses from the nerves causing pain. You may have these procedures tried if you have severe back pain from crushed vertebrae. Ask your primary care doctor to refer you, if nothing else has worked.

Chapter 13

Recovering from a Fracture When You Have Osteoporosis

In This Chapter

- Looking for osteoporosis
- Avoiding falls
- Knowing which bones are most likely to break
- Healing your bones
- Avoiding another fracture

You may not have thought much about osteoporosis — until you fracture a bone. Sad to say, many people aren't diagnosed with or treated for osteoporosis until after they've sustained their first fracture.

This is especially true if you don't fall into the stereotypical osteoporosis; for example, older men, who do have osteoporosis in significant numbers (see Chapter 4 for more on men and osteoporosis), may not even consider the possibility because they think osteoporosis is a "woman's disease."

We're hoping you're reading this book *before* you've broken a bone, not while you're resting on the floor waiting for someone to come and find you after a fall. All kidding aside, a broken bone is no laughing matter, and our goal is to prevent as many broken bones as possible.

However, some fractures may occur, and we want you to know what to expect if you have one. If you suffer any of the fractures we discuss in this chapter, have your doctor thoroughly evaluate you for causes of osteoporosis. Then you can work together to proactively prevent your next break.

In this chapter, we discuss how to prevent breaking bones in the first place, which bones are most likely to fracture, what type of treatment you're likely to undergo, and how you can get through it with — well, maybe not a smile on your face, but with a minimum of discomfort and inconvenience.

Checking for Osteoporosis after a Fracture

Anyone who has had a fragility fracture, such as a hip fracture, spontaneous break of a bone in their back, or a wrist fracture (see Chapter 1 for more on fragility fractures) needs to be evaluated for osteoporosis or some other cause of weak bones, such as osteomalacia. This workup may include bone density measurements (see Chapter 9) and blood testing.

Anyone who has continued back pain, or who has lost several inches of height, needs to be evaluated to see if his or her height loss is due to *compression fractures,* fractures of the vertebrae. (See "Comprehending vertebral compression fractures" later in this chapter for the lowdown on compression fractures.)

Preventing Falls

Clearly, avoiding falls is an obvious defense against broken bones. Unfortunately, falls are a part of many older people's lives.

Falls however are much more than an embarrassing moment or a minor inconvenience. Almost 8,500 people in the United States older than 65 die from injuries sustained in a fall each year. In one study, 25 to 35 percent of adults older than 65 fell once or twice a year, often without being able to pinpoint a reason for the fall.

Even being in a controlled environment, like a nursing home under supervision, doesn't prevent all falls. Approximately 50 percent of nursing home residents fall at least once a year, and 11 percent of those who fall seriously injure themselves. By comparison, 30 percent of seniors living independently fall each year, more than half in their own homes.

As you age, your risk of falling increases. Around 50 percent of people older than age 80 fall at least once each year (these falls aren't all attributed to osteoporosis). Why so many falls when you get older? The causes are many, but some of the biggest offenders are

- Confusion
- Dizziness/vertigo
- Hearing problems
- Joint problems such as osteoarthritis involving lumbar spine, hip, or knee
- Low blood pressure
- Multiple medications/sedating medications
- Poor balance
- Poor eyesight
- Unsteady *gait* (pattern of walking)
- Weakness from previous stroke

Preventing all falls may be impossible, but you can prevent a large number by taking a few simple precautions. To decrease your chance of falling, try these suggestions:

- Put grab bars in the bathtub or shower and use them.
- Clear clutter from your house, and don't change your furniture around too often!
- Light your house well.
- Wear nonskid socks or slippers.
- When you get up out of bed or out of a chair, rise slowly, and have something sturdy nearby to use to steady yourself.
- Make sure your doctor is aware of all the medications you take, even the OTC ones like Benadryl, which can make you sleepy.
- Use handrails when you go up and down stairs, and make sure they're secure. It doesn't help if you *and* the handrail both end up falling down the steps!
- Don't carry heavy loads up or down the steps, like big baskets of laundry. Take smaller loads and make two trips if necessary. Carrying a large load obscures your vision and may also make you unstable.
- Tripping over a sleeping pet is easy. Put something easily visible on your pet, a reflective collar or a very bright ribbon so you can spot her more easily.
- If you use a wheelchair, be careful getting in and out; always check to make sure the brake is locked.
- Get rid of slippery rugs, especially in the bathroom or the kitchen, where the floor is likely to be slippery.

- Keep your steps free of ice and snow; hire a neighbor to do it. It's money well spent.
- Stay off ladders! That goes for climbing on kitchen chairs too. (Now, if only your co-author Sharon could get her mom to do this!)

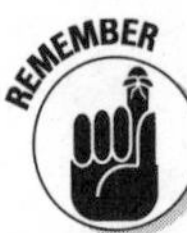

Altering your lifestyle is sometimes difficult. You may feel like you're not independent if you can't do things for yourself, like painting the 8-foot ceilings in your living room. But remember that your independence will decrease even more significantly if you become a fall statistic. So please — don't change the second-story storm windows by yourself!

Recognizing Breaks and What's Most Likely to Break

How do you know if you've broken a bone? Sometimes it's quite obvious; for instance, if you have a compound fracture, the bone is sticking out of the skin! Some fractures aren't so obvious. You should suspect a bone is broken when:

- It hurts to move or touch the broken part.
- The broken part has bruising.
- The arm or leg is shorter than normal, or turns inward or outward.
- You hear a "snap" at the time of the injury.
- You can't put any weight on the broken part.

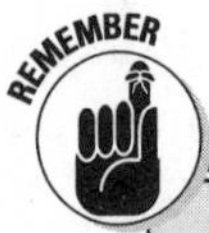

Wearing hip protectors

You may not win any fashion awards with what looks like bulky underwear, but hip protectors with their extra padding placed at the sides can reduce your chance of a hip fracture if you fall.

One downside to hip protectors is that they're expensive; a pair can cost nearly $100. Several brands are available, with names like Safehip, HIPS, and Hip guard.

One of the best Internet sites carries a good selection of sizes and brands, as well as selling other aids to help you live fall free. Check out `www.hiprotector.com`. In addition to selling several brands of hip protectors, the site also offers medical alert alarms and rails to help you get out of bed without falling.

So are you wondering which types of fractures are the most common with osteoporosis? If you experience any of these fractures, ask your doctor to check you for osteoporosis. If you already have osteoporosis, be vigilant about preventing these breaks:

- **Hip fractures:** Although hip fractures may seem to get the most publicity with osteoporosis, they aren't the most common osteoporotic fracture. Of the 1.5 million osteoporotic fractures each year in the United States, approximately 300,000 are hip fractures.
- **Vertebral compression fractures:** Nearly half, or 700,000, of the annual osteoporotic fractures in the United States are vertebral compression fractures.
- **Wrist fractures:** Often called Colles' fractures, these types account for about 200,000 of the annual osteoporotic fractures in the United States.
- **Other fractures:** The remainder includes mostly fractures of the ribs, shoulder, and pelvis, although any bone can sustain an osteoporotic fracture.

Although vertebral compression fractures can occur with little or no trauma — a cough or sudden twist of your upper body can cause one — hip and wrist fractures are most often related to falls. The following sections detail each type of fracture and the specifics you need to know.

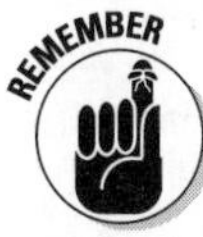

If you decrease your chance of falling, you decrease your chance of fracture. Make sure you're doing all you can to stay on your feet and off the floor! (Check out "Preventing Falls" earlier in this chapter for specific ways to avoid falling.)

Handling hip fractures

Despite your best efforts to improve your bone strength and avoid falls, some of you are going to fracture your hip. In fact, many of you — men and women — will sustain a hip fracture — 300,000 of you each year.

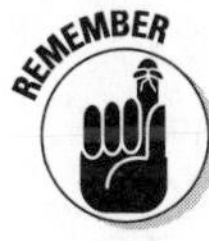

Hip fractures usually make it difficult, if not impossible, for you to walk, but some people with a fracture have only vague pain in their back, buttocks, groin, or thighs, and can walk normally. Some fractures cause shortening of one leg with the foot and knee pointing outwards.

Because joints and muscles are often sore in people older than 65, determining whether a fracture is present, or if the pain has another cause, such as osteoarthritis, is important. If you even just suspect that you may have a fracture, get treatment as quickly as possible, to prevent complications. Most hip fractures are easily seen on plain radiographs (X-ray) although some are seen only with a Magnetic Resonance Imaging (MRI) or Computed Tomography (CT) scan, which are specialized highly detailed images of bone.

Where your hip fracture is located is critical. A break can occur in several different places in the femur. Doctors classify the breaks as the following:

- **Intracapsular fractures:** Nearly half of all hip fractures in the elderly are in the femoral neck, and are sometimes called *intracapsular fractures.* They occur one to two inches away from the hip joint.

  Femoral neck fractures can be harder to pin together, because the bone at the break is more fragile and isn't well anchored by the pins. Femoral neck fractures can also disrupt blood flow to the femoral head and can lead to bone death and joint collapse (called *avascular necrosis*).
- **Extracapsular fractures:** These fractures, also called *intertrochanteric* fractures, are lower on the femur.
- Around 55 percent of osteoporotic hip fractures are extracapsular. Other types of extracapsular fractures are *trocanteric* and *subtrocanteric.*

Repairing your hip joint

Hip fractures are usually treated surgically. Some require total hip replacement, while others can be pinned together and allowed to heal. It depends on where the break is and how much "good" bone your surgeon has to work with.

If your fracture is at the neck of the femur, just below the ball and socket joint (an intracapsular break), your doctor may recommend putting in a prosthetic metal hip joint, also called *arthroplasty.* This procedure is often necessary in older patients because the broken area won't have enough blood supply to heal well, and may develop *osteonecrosis,* or, literally, "dead bone." The dead section of bone will eventually weaken and collapse.

If both the ball and the hip socket are replaced, it's called a total hip replacement. If only the ball is replaced, it's a partial hip replacement (*hemiathroplasty*). Hip replacement parts generally last 10 to 15 years.

Your new hip can be fixed to bone in several ways. Some prosthetic devices are attached to the bone with rapidly setting plastic cement called *methyl methacrylate.* Others are held in place by bone growing directly into a roughened coating on the prosthesis.

Each type of fixation has its advantages and disadvantages. An uncemented prosthesis may last longer in some people, because there's no cement to fail under repeated loading over the years. On the downside, recovery can take longer with an uncemented prosthesis, because it takes time for bone to attach and grow into the prosthesis. You may have to limit activities for as long as three months. And you're also more likely to have pain in the thigh as the new bone grows.

Cemented replacements are used more frequently than cementless ones for patients with osteoporosis or those with weakened bones. Sometimes surgeons perform a hybrid procedure, where they cement one component and not the other.

Fractures that occur lower on the neck of the femur (extracapsular fractures) have a couple options. The surgeon can fix them internally by pinning the broken area back together with a surgical plate and screws or pins, or the surgeon can perform a hip replacement.

Preparing yourself for surgery and aftercare

Your doctor will probably have a printed list of what to expect after your surgery if your surgery is planned ahead of time. However, it never hurts to hear everything twice, especially when going into the hospital for major surgery.

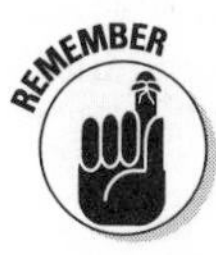

Sometimes your doctor will perform the surgery shortly after your hip fracture, and you won't have time to square everything away. You may have to rely on your spouse, a friend, or relative to get everything in order for your discharge home. This simple list can get them started:

1. **Plan to have someone stay with you for a few weeks, if you live alone.**

   You aren't going to be anywhere near as mobile as you hope you're going to be. Recovering from surgery is difficult, and having someone to save you steps can be a big benefit. Try to progress your activities as much as your surgeon allows.

2. **Rent crutches or a walker if your hospital doesn't provide them.**

   You may find it easier to start with a walker, especially because you can attach a carry bag to the walker with all your essentials. Depending on the type of person you are, these essentials could include the latest paperback, knitting or crocheting material, or the TV remote! You'll probably want to keep your glasses, tissues, medications, telephone, and possibly a water bottle with you as well. Buy a big bag, but make sure it hangs evenly off the front of the walker; you don't want extra weight pulling from either side.

You may feel much more stable using a walker for the first few days or weeks; crutches can be hard to manage. After you graduate to crutches, wear a carpenter's apron (or a frilly apron, if you prefer!) or something with big pockets to carry your essential items around.

3. **Clear a path through your frequently used rooms.**

   You may be surprised at how many small rugs and pieces of furniture you find in your way when you get home. You used to sidestep them without a second thought, but now they can be major obstacles to getting around without another fall.

4. **Arrange a downstairs sleeping area.**

   If all your bedrooms are on the second floor, you may want to rent a hospital bed. Getting on and off a low couch may be difficult or not recommended by your surgeon.

5. **Check your bathroom for accessibility to the toilet.**

   Some bathrooms are rather cramped and you may find it difficult, if not impossible, to maneuver your walker close enough to ease yourself onto the toilet.

   If maneuvering around your bathroom looks to be a problem, rent a portable toilet. These rented johns are usually higher than a standard toilet and easier to get onto when you're using a walker or crutches.

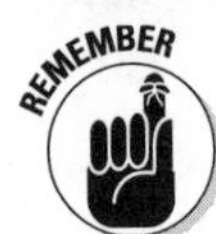

   You may also want to consider your shower setup. Showers seats are available so you can sit comfortably while taking a shower. A hand-held shower nozzle can make washing your hair easier. Getting down into a bathtub may be difficult for several months after surgery. Your doctor may even recommend against using a bathtub.

6. **Don't plan on cooking any big dinners.**

   Forget about cooking Thanksgiving dinner for your clan of 20. The turkey can wait! Let someone else host this year. In addition, have a good supply of frozen dinners on hand, or else make sure the person staying with you doesn't mind doing the cooking.

What to expect at the hospital

If you've never had surgery before, you may not know what to expect. Although procedures may vary somewhat from hospital to hospital, most will follow this pattern:

1. **Your doctor will discuss your surgery with you and have you sign a surgical consent.**

   A nurse may also give you pain medication if you're uncomfortable. Some recent studies have shown that patients whose hip surgery is performed within 24 hours of the fracture have less pain. Sometimes surgery can't be done that quickly if you have other medical issues that need medical clearance before surgery.

2. **You may have an electrocardiogram (EKG) done and blood drawn to assess your general health and look for any potential problems, such as anemia or an infection.**

   Some hip fractures can result in considerable loss of blood even before surgery.

3. **The anesthesiologist may come in to discuss anesthesia with you.**

   Your doctor can perform hip surgery under general or regional anesthesia, like a spinal or epidural. A review of several recent studies shows that regional anesthesia may be slightly more beneficial for hip surgery. But you may experience more pain while the anesthesiologist is administering the anesthesia because you'll need to be rolled on your side.

   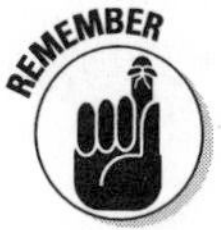

   You won't be allowed to eat or drink anything for 12 hours or so before surgery so that your stomach is empty and the risk of aspiration during surgery will be decreased. *Aspiration* occurs when the contents of your stomach move up into the throat and down into your lungs. Sounds ugly and it is!

4. **You'll be taken down to a preoperative area to wait for your surgery.**

   If you don't already have an intravenous line (IV), a nurse will put one into your vein. The surgery lasts approximately two to three hours. You may have a 10-to-12-inch incision if you had standard hip surgery; if you have minimal incision surgery, you'll have a 3-to-5-inch incision.

5. **You'll be taken after surgery to a recovery area, where you'll remain until you're awake and your vital signs, like your blood pressure and heart rate, are stable.**

   You'll probably be in the recovery area for an hour or so. A nurse will frequently check your blood pressure and pulse. As soon as your vital signs are stable, you'll be moved to your room.

6. **The day after surgery, you'll be encouraged to sit up and possibly even stand for a short period.**

   Doing so helps keep blood clots from developing.

Getting back on your feet without complications

Because there's a high risk for complications after hip surgery, your doctor will want you back on your feet as soon as possible — probably much sooner than you feel like getting up!

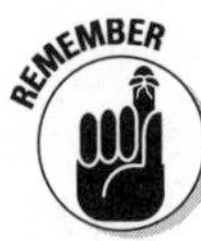

You may find yourself on your feet with the help of a walker or crutches just a few days after surgery. Moving around is crucial to keep you from developing pneumonia or blood clots from staying in bed too long.

You'll probably spend less than seven days in the hospital after a hip pinning replacement. After the initial time in the hospital, you may go home or spend a few days or few weeks in a rehabilitation center for further recovery. In the rehab center you'll spend your days under the watchful eyes of specially trained therapists, nurses, and physicians. When you're discharged home depends on a number of factors, such as your overall general health and whether or not you have anyone to help you after you get home.

If you have a hip replacement, the most common postoperative complication is a hip dislocation. Essentially, the ball slips out of the socket.

To avoid dislocation, don't place your hip in certain positions, such as pulling your knees up to your chest, or crossing your affected leg past the midline of your body. Your hip becomes dislocated because the artificial ball and socket need time for scar tissue to stabilize the hip. The ball can become dislodged from the socket more easily during the first three months after surgery.

As with any surgery, you can develop an infection at the surgical site. Your doctor probably will prescribe antibiotics to help prevent infection. You may also need to do breathing exercises for the first few days to keep your lungs working well so you don't develop pneumonia.

Over the long term, foreign material in your body can cause an inflammatory reaction. This can happen after hip replacement surgery when small pieces of material wear off the artificial joint and are absorbed by surrounding tissue. The inflammation can eventually result in bone destruction near the implant, causing it to become loose. Check with your surgeon about yearly visits for early detection of this problem.

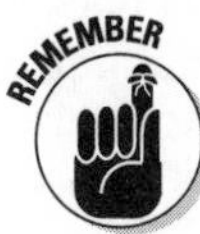

Because problems with infection deep within the bone can occur years after your surgery, tell your dentist or doctor before having any procedures done, even teeth cleaning. They may want to prescribe prophylactic antibiotics.

Because of the risk of developing blood clots (also known as *deep vein thrombosis,* or DVT) due to decreased mobility and damage to the veins during surgery, you may be given a blood thinner, such as aspirin, warfarin (Coumadin), or heparin, at the time of surgery and for a short time afterwards. Newer types of blood thinners known as fondapiranux are also available.

Your doctor may also ask you to wear compression stockings. These stockings keep the blood flow moving through your legs to help avoid clot development.

Physical activity after hip replacement

Early mobility is the key to recovering from hip surgery. Getting back on your feet helps you avoid certain complications like blood clots and pneumonia, which actually cause more mortality than the surgeries themselves.

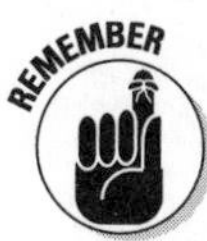

Having a new hip joint may tempt you to try to become more physically active. Remember that physical exercise is good for you. It can reduce joint pain and stiffness and increase muscle and bone strength. However, don't forget that artificial hip joints have a more limited range of motion than your original hip joint, so you may need to discover new ways to sit or bend to avoid damaging the joint.

Your doctor may discourage activities that put high-impact stress on your hip joint, such as running, basketball, or tennis. Walking or swimming are low-impact exercises that can help improve muscle strength, although swimming doesn't increase bone strength because it's a nonweight-bearing activity (see Chapter 6 for more on exercise).

Your doctor will probably prescribe physical therapy after your surgery (see the following section), and you can be assured that your physical therapist will assess your recovery carefully and will start with simple activity before moving on to more demanding routines.

Therapy after hip surgery

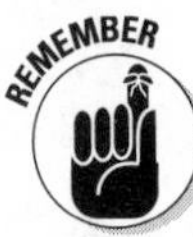

Physical therapy is critically important in osteoporosis, because bed rest can lead to more bone loss. However, getting back to normal after any fracture isn't easy. With hip surgery, getting back to normal is even more difficult. Statistics show that less than half of those people who undergo hip surgery ever regain their former mobility or quality of life.

We don't provide these stats to discourage you, but to motivate you. You can regain a great deal of your former abilities with physical therapy, but it'll take work. The more you know about what will help you get back to whatever is "normal" for you, the better equipped you'll be for the demands of the post-surgery period. (See Chapter 12 for more on pain management after a broken bone.)

Many doctors recommend physical therapy after most kinds of injuries and orthopedic surgeries. Physical therapists are specially trained to develop an exercise regimen specific to you. First, they assess your abilities. Then they work with you to increase the difficulty of your exercise program as you become stronger.

You may feel as though you're barely out of anesthesia before physical and occupational therapists (under the guidance of a physician specializing in rehabilitation medicine) are in your room, encouraging you to get moving. (Occupational therapists are specialized therapists trained in rehabilitation of upper extremity problems.) You can check out the sidebar, "Encountering two therapists — physical and occupational," in this chapter for more on what therapists do.

Encountering two therapists — physical and occupational

Physical therapists and occupational therapists are both specially trained professionals who have advanced degrees and are integral parts of the healthcare team when it comes to musculoskeletal problems. Both help people improve their ability to perform tasks in their daily living and working environments.

Physical therapists do much more than take care of patients after osteoporotic fractures. They may take care of accident victims and people with disabilities, such as low-back pain, arthritis, heart disease, head injuries, and cerebral palsy.

A physical therapist may help you if you have had surgery by

- Helping you develop or regain strength and flexibility
- Working to develop pain control techniques
- Improving your balance and coordination
- Decreasing swelling and inflammation in joints

Meanwhile, occupational therapists help individuals with physical, mental, or emotional handicaps to develop, recover, or maintain daily living and work skills. Some are specially trained to look at the small joints of the hand and wrist. They create custom braces to protect hand joints that are damaged by injury or arthritis.

An occupational therapist may help you if you have had surgery by

- Assessing your home for falling hazards
- Helping you modify your environment to decrease the chance of injury
- Protect your upper extremities from injury when using a cane or walker

An occupational therapist also often manages rehabilitation after a wrist fracture.

In your first sessions, your physical therapist works at getting you to move safely in and out of bed, without doing damage to yourself. You'll also discover how to properly use a walker or crutches. An occupational therapist may help you with figuring out how to get dressed and bathed.

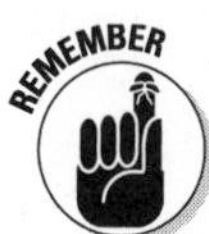

If you go to a rehab hospital after surgery, you'll discover how to gradually do your daily care yourself, and as time progresses, to walk farther and with fewer physical aids, a single point cane, and finally to just your own two feet!

You may not be back to your own two feet when you graduate from the rehabilitation facility, though. Up to 85 percent of patients are still using a cane or other device for walking six months after their fracture. Have your doctor evaluate you after six months or so to make sure your recovery is on track.

Make sure you eat well. Eating well is a critical part of healing from a hip fracture. Plenty of protein (20 grams per day) and supplementation of calcium and vitamin D have been proven to increase your bone mineral density and speed your recovery. See Chapter 5 for more on nutrition.

If you need revision surgery . . .

Only around 10 percent of hip surgeries need to be revised or redone over a five-to-ten-year period, but if you're one of the 10 percent, that statistic isn't going to make you feel any better.

Doctors have to perform revision surgery for a number of reasons:

- *Aseptic loosening* is the most common, where the hip implants become loose within the bone. This loosening can be painful.
- Wear of the polyethylene-bearing surface in the socket
- A break of the prosthesis
- A break in the bone around the prosthesis
- Infection

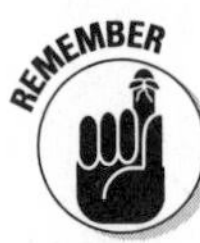

Revision surgery is more complicated than the first hip surgery, for several reasons. The bone around the implant may be in poor condition to attach to, and removing the prosthesis may necessitate more extensive surgery. Also, the unfortunate fact is that you're probably going to be older at the time of revision surgery than you were at the time of the original surgery. Age brings more problems with mobility and increased chance of complications.

However, don't worry too much about revision surgery. Knowing how long, on average, a hip replacement lasts can be reassuring. The following list shows how long hip replacements last, on average:

After ten years, 90 percent of hip replacements still function well.

After 20 years, around 80 percent still function well.

After 25 to 30 years, around 50 percent still function well.

Comprehending vertebral compression fractures

Some of you reading this book already have vertebral compression fractures and don't know it. Around 25 percent of all postmenopausal women in the United States have at least one; if you're a postmenopausal woman older than 80, your odds increase to 40 percent. (See Chapter 12 for more about vertebral compression fractures.)

Vertebral compression fractures occur when the weight of your upper body exceeds the ability of your spine to support the load. Ironically, you're more likely to have a spinal fracture if you're small. Overweight people are less likely to have vertebral compression fractures, probably because their weight-bearing load is increased, which strengthens their bones.

The two common types of osteoporotic spinal fractures are

- **Wedge fractures:** In a wedge fracture, part of the vertebral body collapses, making the bone into the shape of a wedge. If several vertebral bodies collapse, the spine bends forward, which is called *kyphosis* (see Chapter 7 for more about kyphosis).
- **Burst fractures:** In a burst fracture, the break goes all the way across the vertebrae, causing loss of height.

Both wedge fractures and burst fractures can cause a number of complications. These complications include

- Bowel obstruction
- Chronic pain
- Constipation
- Crowding of internal organs
- Decreased self esteem
- Loss of height
- Loss of urine control
- Respiratory disease
- Weight loss due to abdominal compression

Diagnosing compression fractures

Only about a third of vertebral fractures are diagnosed, partly because back pain is considered by many to be a normal part of aging, and also because some vertebral compression fractures don't cause pain.

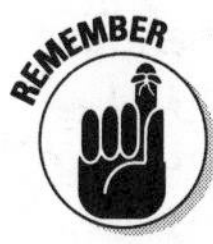

The standard method for diagnosing compression fractures is X-ray. Make sure your doctor orders pictures of the lumbar and thoracic spines from both front and side views. Statistics show that up to 20 percent of people have more than one compression fracture present.

A CT scan can help diagnose fractures not easily seen on X-ray. A CT scan can also diagnose burst fractures that may appear to be wedge fractures on X-ray (see the previous section about the differences between wedge and burst fractures). An MRI is recommended if your doctor suspects spinal cord compression or other neurological involvement.

Compression fractures can occur anywhere on your spinal column, although they're seen most commonly in certain vertebrae, namely T8 through 12, L1, and L4. For more information about the different parts of your spine, visit `www.back.com/anatomy.html`.

Treating compression fractures

Treatment for compression fractures runs the gamut. Depending on the location and symptoms of your fracture, your doctor can do the following:

- **Bed rest and painkillers:** If you have a stable fracture, one that won't be displaced by movement, your doctor may simply prescribe a few days' rest and mild painkillers, if necessary (see Chapter 12 for more on pain medication for fractures). *Calcitonin,* a hormone sometimes used to help prevent bone fractures, can also help decrease pain from vertebral compression fractures.
- **Brace:** Your doctor can also prescribe a bracing device called a Thoracic-Lumbar-Sacral Orthosis (TLSO) to treat a spinal fracture. Some doctors prefer not to use bracing, however, because using constant support may weaken your bone.

  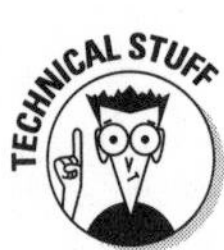

  To make TLSO a little easier to understand, the term *thoracic* refers to your chest area, *lumbar* and *sacral* your lower back.

  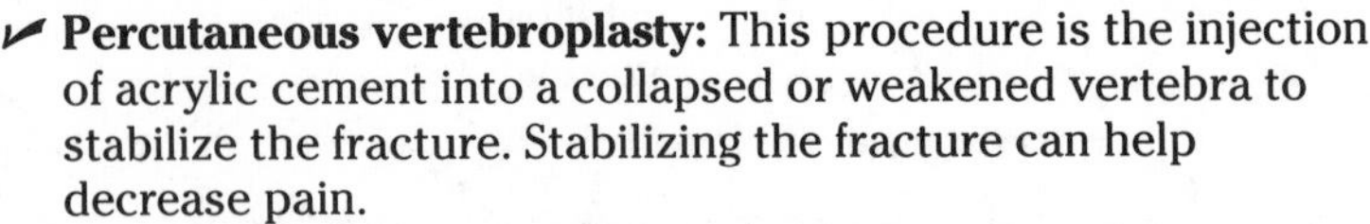
- **Percutaneous vertebroplasty:** This procedure is the injection of acrylic cement into a collapsed or weakened vertebra to stabilize the fracture. Stabilizing the fracture can help decrease pain.

  You'll probably be sedated with an IV medication or other sedative during the procedure. If you have severe pain, you may need general anesthesia for the procedure, because it may be too painful for you to stay lying down in the position necessary to inject the cement.

  After the procedure, you'll need to lie flat for one hour to allow the cement to harden. You may need to stay in the hospital for another hour or so for observation, at which time you should be able to stand and walk. It may take up to three days to feel pain relief, although some people have immediate relief.
- **Kyphoplasty:** This technique is new for stabilizing vertebral fractures and decreasing pain. Kyphoplasty is done through a small incision in the back under either a local or general anesthetic, depending upon the severity of the case. The entire procedure takes about an hour for each treated vertebra. You should be in the hospital no longer than a day; you may possibly be allowed to return home the same day. You may notice pain relief within two days of surgery.

The advantage of kyphoplasty over vertebroplasty is that kyphoplasty may return the spine to a more normal alignment, decreasing the dreaded "dowager's hump."

Pain relief was reported in more than 90 percent of kyphoplasty patients. However, the new technique is still in its infancy. Only about 500 patients have received this treatment. Complications occur in about 1 percent of individuals and can be mild or serious. Allergic reactions to the cement have been reported, and the most serious complications are bleeding related to needle placement and damage to a nerve or the spinal cord.

Recovering from vertebral compression fractures

If you have spinal compression fractures, you may be in a great deal of pain and not be able to move around much at first. However, as soon as possible, provided that you don't have damage to the nerves in your back, you need to engage in a physical therapy program.

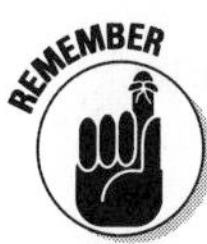

Don't spend too much time in bed, because prolonged bed rest weakens bone. Get up as soon as possible, even if you can only stay up for short periods of 30 to 60 minutes at a time.

Work to begin walking as soon as possible, being careful to maintain good posture, which helps reduce the load on the fracture and decrease pain. You can start with walking for just a few minutes and work up gradually to 20 minutes or so by adding a minute or two each week.

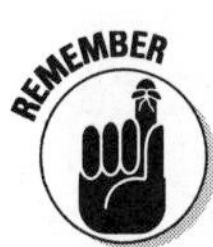

Exercise is important after a vertebral fracture, but it needs to be the right type of exercise. Until your fracture is healed, usually within 8 to 12 weeks, stick to exercises that don't put any strain on your spine, such as sit-ups or toe touches. You can safely strengthen your abdominal muscles just by tightening them as long as you don't move your back.

Ideally you'll have the help of a physical therapist to show you which exercises are safe after a spinal fracture, because the chance of another fracture is high. If you don't already have a therapist, ask your doctor to recommend one.

You may find walking with the help of a rolling walker that has four wheels easier than a walker with the standard two wheels in the front. Avoid standard walkers because you put extra strain on the fractured area each time you lift the walker.

If you have difficulty maintaining good posture, a back brace may help you temporarily. Occupational therapists can help fit you for a back brace, as well as show you the best way to carry out daily activities without putting strain of the fracture.

Want another option? *T'ai Chi,* an ancient eastern practice, is a popular exercise regimen that improves balance and strengthens muscles. Ask your physical therapist if T'ai Chi is right for you! (You can also check out *T'ai Chi For Dummies* by Therese Iknoian and Manny Fuentes [Wiley] for more information.)

With a snap of your wrist — a Colles' fracture

A *Colles' fracture* — the medical term for a wrist fracture — is the result of a normal instinct — the instinct to put your hand out when you're falling, to break your fall.

You may suspect a Colles' fracture if you have pain and swelling just above the wrist, and you can't hold anything with any weight in your hand. The wrist may be at an odd angle to your hand. X-rays can also diagnose a Colles' fracture.

You'll probably need to have the bones realigned and the wrist splinted or casted to keep the bones in proper position to heal. If you've broken more than one bone in the wrist, your doctor may need to pin or otherwise internally immobilize the broken areas.

A Colles' fracture can lead to some loss of mobility in the wrist; you can also have chronic pain if you've injured ligaments in the wrist. You may also develop arthritis or *carpal tunnel syndrome,* a painful compression of a nerve in your wrist, from damage to the median nerve.

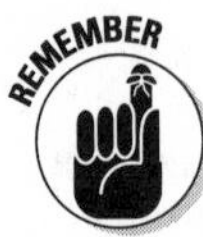

Although a wrist fracture may not seem as serious at first as a hip fracture or spinal fracture, it can be a difficult fracture to recover from. You never know how much you use your wrist until you lose the use of it! In fact, it can take up to two years to fully recover use of your wrist after a fracture, and even then some problems with mobility and pain may remain.

After a wrist fracture, your wrist will be immobilized for six to ten weeks in a cast or splint. You may need to elevate your arm to reduce swelling. Occupational and physical therapy can help you to increase your use of the wrist, helping strengthen it and increase mobility.

Other kinds of fractures

Although hip, spine, and wrist fractures are the most common fractures in osteoporosis, other bones can break too. For example, ribs can break with bouts of coughing or even from an overenthusiastic hug from a grandchild!

Broken ribs are painful, and take between three to eight weeks to heal. You may feel pain especially when taking a deep breath, and may feel better when you "splint" the rib by holding your hand over it. You may also experience some bruising.

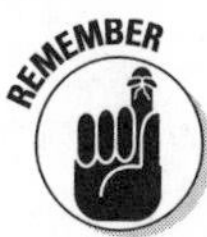

Applying heat to the painful area may help it feel better. Don't wear a binder unless your doctor specifically recommends one. You need to be able to take deep breaths to keep your lungs clear.

The pelvic bones can break as well, usually after a fall. If you fracture your pelvis, you may have pain in your groin, hip, or lower back. Other symptoms may include

- Abdominal pain
- Bleeding from the vagina, *urethra* (urine tube), or rectum
- Difficulty urinating
- Difficulty walking or standing
- Numbness/tingling in the groin or legs

Treatment of pelvic fractures depends on the severity of the break. In the case of a minor fracture, bed rest and OTC or prescription painkillers may be all the treatment needed. Your doctor may also recommend physical therapy, the use of crutches, and surgery. Healing from a pelvic fracture can take anywhere from a few weeks to several months.

How Long Does Bone Take to Heal?

Bone is a complicated living tissue, and its complexity is obvious when you look at the healing process of bone. Exactly how fast the bone heals depends somewhat on what type of bone is broken.

You basically have two types of bone. (See Chapter 2 for more on different types of bone.)

- **Cortical (compact):** Cortical bone is denser, about four to six times denser than trabecular bone. About 75 to 80 percent of your skeleton is made of cortical bone. Cortical bone makes up most of the shafts of long bones, like the femur.

  Cortical bone heals in four to eight months.

- **Trabecular (spongy):** Trabecular bone is spongier and makes up the other 20 percent of bone. Trabecular bone is found at the end of long bones and in the bones of the vertebrae.

  Trabecular bone heals within three to six months. Trabecular bone heals more quickly than cortical bone in part because of its better blood supply.

If you have a problem with low amounts of vitamin D in your blood or some other problem with vitamin D metabolism, it will take much longer for your fracture to heal. (See Chapter 11 for information on vitamin D.)

Reducing the Chance of Another Fracture

Statistics show that if you've had one osteoporotic fracture, your chances for another one increase. After you know your bones are more prone to fracture, you need to be extra vigilant about taking care of yourself. Now is the time to intervene.

Make sure that you receive follow-up from your primary care doctor or rheumatologist. Take your medications (Chapter 12), exercise regularly (Chapter 6), eat well (Chapter 5), take your calcium and vitamin D supplements (Chapter 11), and don't hang off second-story ladders.

Chapter 14

Focusing on the Future of Osteoporosis

In This Chapter

- Expanding prevention
- Improving diagnosis
- Uncovering new meds
- Relying on new surgical techniques
- Combating osteoporosis worldwide
- Looking at the next generation

When Dr. O'Connor first started studying *rheumatology* (the study of bones and joints), there was no good way to detect early osteoporosis. In fact, no medications were even available to improve fragile bone. Fortunately with the advancements of science, a simple testing procedure has been developed to detect early bone disease. Doctors also now have treatments, that when instituted early, can build bone density.

In this chapter, we show that even though the medical field has come a long way, it still has many challenges ahead in eradicating osteoporosis and making everyone's bones as strong as Superman's (or Superwoman's).

Improving Osteoporosis Prevention

Recent research has identified the burden of bone disease, which is staggering, not only in terms of money spent, but also in terms of problems that can't be as easily measured such as loss of independence.

Scientists can predict the number of fractures and costs of those fractures if nothing is done to change the current trend. Doctors and researchers also have the tools, such as diagnosis and medications, to decrease osteoporosis in the next generation.

Unfortunately, just having the information doesn't always change things. For example, doctors know that changing diet and exercise patterns in girls between the ages of 9 and 12 makes a difference in their adult bone strength. The challenge is to translate that information into changes that truly alter the face of osteoporosis forever.

How do doctors encourage patients to change habits?

You probably know how difficult it is to change established habits. Almost everyone knows that smoking, drinking excessively, and lying on the couch eating bon bons all day isn't healthy, but people still do them. So how do doctors change habits, not only individually, but also nationwide? We suggest these ideas:

- Doctors can discover lessons learned from other health education campaigns such as those campaigns that promote smoking cessation.
- Doctors can educate through population-based approaches.
- Doctors can educate one-on-one.

Research needs to be done to investigate which interventions are most effective in changing behaviors. What messages are most effective for children? What messages work better for men?

We hope that the readers of this book will not only improve their own bone health, but will also take the steps to improve the bone health of their family members.

Relying on professional associations

Several major organizations have missions solely directed toward improving bone health. They're constantly working to increase knowledge of how osteoporosis can be prevented. The most notable organizations are the American Society for Bone and Mineral Research (www.asbmr.org), the National Osteoporosis Foundation (www.nof.org), and the American College of Rheumatology (www.rheumatology.org).

How are healthcare providers educated?

Healthcare providers realistically can't know every detail about every topic in medicine. Through writing this book and reading literature and seeing patients, your authors have become experts in this field. However, no physician could possibly know every detail about bone disease. But if the majority of healthcare providers understood some key facts about osteoporosis and then implemented them, it could result in a major improvement in the quality of many people's bones.

For example, about five years ago, a study in Pennsylvania showed that only 20 percent of patients who had a hip fracture ever filled a prescription for a drug that was known to improve bone density. Although some of those patients might not have filled a prescription that was given to them by their doctors, many more probably never even received a prescription for an osteoporosis medication.

Other studies have shown that too few patients with a *fragility fracture,* a bone that breaks with minimal or no trauma, were consequently worked up with a DXA scan or with medication.

What could be the causes for this lack of doctor and patient follow-up? Here are some possibilities:

- When patients break a bone and then the fracture heals, they may think they don't need any further treatment, especially if their doctor doesn't stress the need for follow-up.
- Many people fail to understand the connection between fragility fractures and osteoporosis. (See Chapter 1 for more on fragility fractures.)
- Coordination of patient care among several doctors could result in no one taking the responsibility of initiating treatment for osteoporosis. (This is the proverbial "someone needs to take the ball and run with it" problem!)

  For example, your family doctor may think your gynecologist is looking after your osteoporosis — or vice versa.
- Healthcare providers may feel that starting treatment in patients who are older would be too difficult and complicated.
- The doctor or patient might feel that osteoporosis medications won't work, because a fracture has already occurred.

Clearly, understanding why certain patients with osteoporosis don't get treated can improve strategies to identify those people at risk.

The hospital where Dr. O'Connor practices has initiated a program to alert residents in training to initiate a "fragility fracture workup" when a patient is admitted to the hospital with a fracture that could be due to osteoporosis or another metabolic bone disease. A fragility fracture typically is a hip, spine, or wrist fracture and is related to lack of bone strength.

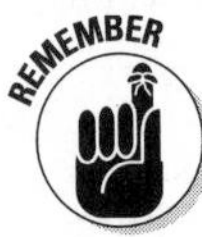

Initiating this type of evaluation is a step in the right direction. When encountering a patient with a fracture, every doctor needs to reflect on whether or not her patient has experienced a fracture with minimal trauma. If the doctor suspects a fragility fracture, then she needs to order the appropriate testing to determine whether osteoporosis or osteomalacia is present. (*Osteomalacia* is soft bones due to problems in making mineral deposit on bone. See Chapter 1 for more on the differences between osteoporosis and osteomalacia.) Then the doctor needs to ask: Why does my patient have osteoporosis?

Needing more research in prevention

There's no question that preventing bone loss before it occurs is better than trying to play catch up and strengthen bone that has already become weakened.

In Chapter 1, we describe how you achieve your highest bone density in your 20s and 30s. Ideally you want to have a high bone density in your early adulthood, because the higher your peak bone mineral density, the more bone you can lose before you fall into the dangerous, fracture-prone range. Research has shown that exercise and calcium intake are two key factors that increase peak bone mineral density. But much more research is needed regarding what other factors determine peak bone mineral density.

A great deal of attention has recently been focused on vitamin D deficiency in the elderly (see Chapters 5 and 11 for more on vitamin D deficiency). Would the use of more vitamin D supplementation in food be the solution? Or would it be preferable to encourage everyone to have their vitamin D level measured after age 55? This screening blood test would follow the pattern of many other tests that are performed routinely for prevention. Many of you already check your cholesterol, thyroid, blood count, and PSA (a test for possible prostate cancer) every year. Testing blood for vitamin D levels wouldn't be difficult.

Only in the last few years has emphasis shifted from calcium alone to calcium plus vitamin D as essential for bone maintenance. Research into vitamin D and bone health indicates that current published guidelines for adequate circulating levels of circulating vitamin D may be woefully low. Doctors and their patients still need more information regarding how much vitamin D is required for adequate bone mineralization throughout growth and development.

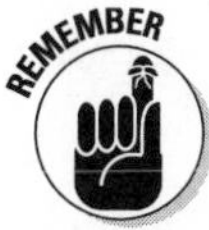

In this book, we increase the recommended daily amount of Vitamin D to 800 IU in people older than 70.

Looking at Future Technologies for Your Bones

Researchers are continuously working to develop new technologies to look inside the human body and analyze the DNA codes that make you *you*. We hope the technology of the next decade will make it possible not only to diagnose and treat osteoporosis in its earliest stages, but also to predict who will have osteoporosis and give preventive treatment long before any evidence of the disease develops.

Better diagnosing for fragile bone

The current definition of osteoporosis depends in large part upon a radiological technique, called Dual Energy X-Ray Absorptiometry (DXA), which has certain technical limitations. In 1990, researchers interested in bone disease met in Copenhagen, Denmark, and defined osteoporosis as "a disease of bony fragility, characterized by low bone mass, micro architectural deterioration of bone tissue and a consequent increase in fracture risk." This definition moves away from the idea that osteoporosis is strictly related to a measurement on a DXA scan.

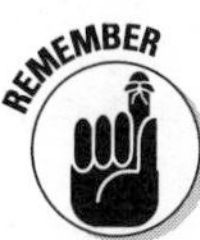

DXA scans only measure bone density in two dimensions. Researchers are developing new radiological techniques that can better analyze bone architecture. Using sophisticated computer programming techniques, radiologists are discovering how to measure bone strength in three dimensions. This technology is referred to as helical or volumetric CT scanning. Some evidence suggests that these types of scans will give a more accurate picture of the precise structure of bone.

Understanding how your genes lead to osteoporosis

In Chapter 3 we mention how important your family history is in predicting your risk for osteoporosis. But just what role does heredity have in determining your peak bone mineral density? And what role does heredity have in determining your rate of bone loss after menopause or *andropause* (male menopause)?

Researchers might be able to answer these questions (and many others) by looking at the genes that are linked to fractures or low bone density. For example, researchers are working on these questions in Iceland, a country where the population is small enough that blood to analyze DNA can be obtained from every single person.

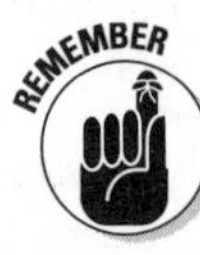

The illness called osteoporosis is really a *heterogeneous disease,* which means that there are different causes of bone loss in different individuals. In other words, your decreased bone strength and your neighbor's low bone strength may have two entirely different causes and may need two entirely different treatments. This makes dissecting the genetic factors very challenging.

Another way of approaching the problem is to look for rare diseases affecting bone density. One such rare disease occurs in children and causes fractures. A researcher has shown that this disease is linked to a defective low-density lipoprotein receptor protein 5 gene. Interestingly, when this gene is overactive, an illness with very high bone density results.

Finding Future Medications

Several effective drugs are now available for treating osteoporosis, but many have side effects that make them difficult or impossible for some women to take.

Because some of the drugs available have to be taken daily, there's a potential for noncompliance, with some people not taking their medication due to confusion or just plain forgetfulness. Some new medications can be taken less frequently, or by intermittent intravenous infusion.

New ways of giving bisphosphonates

As we discuss in Chapter 10, one of the side effects of bisphosphonates is *esophagitis,* an irritation of the esophagus. Therefore if you have a problem with your esophagus, your doctor might not allow you to take alendronate or risedronate.

If you do have esophagitis, your doctor may consider intravenous forms of bisphosphonates. One type is pamidronate, which has been used for years for the treatment of Paget's disease and certain complications of metastatic cancer. Dr. O'Connor often uses pamidronate in her patients with esophageal problems.

Unfortunately, the Food and Drug Administration (FDA) hasn't approved pamidronate for use in osteoporosis. Therefore some insurance companies don't pay for its use. Nonetheless, some literature and anecdotal evidence indicates that this medication is safe and effective and it works similarly to other bisphonphonates.

Although pamidronate is administered four times per year, another new disphosphonate has been developed that can be administered once a year. This drug is known as zoledronic acid.

In 2002, a study on zoledronic acid showed that one dose yearly increased bone mineral density. Larger trials with more people and over a longer period of time are underway to assess whether fractures rates can be reduced. (See Chapter 10 for more information about pamidronate and zoledronic acid.)

Experimenting with new synthetic estrogens

A new synthetic estrogen compound, Estren, increased bone density and strength in female and male mice without the side effects associated with hormone replacement therapy (HRT). Although what works in mice doesn't always work in people, Estren could be an alternative treatment for women who stopped using HRT because of the recently uncovered associated risks for cancer and heart disease.

Estren is part of a new class of compounds called ANGELS (Activators of Non-Genomic Estrogen-Like Signaling). Scientists were able to separate estrogen's bone-strengthening chemicals from those that affect the reproductive system. Estren, which contains chemicals that appear to preserve bone mass, didn't cause any side effects in the reproductive tissue of mice. More animal studies will need to be done before Estren is tested on people.

Developing new drug compounds by studying bone biology

Research is ongoing to develop substances that can keep bone producing what it needs to stay strong. One method that researchers are developing for improving bone density in people with osteoporosis is looking for substances that prevent *osteoclasts* (cells that break down bone) from binding to bone.

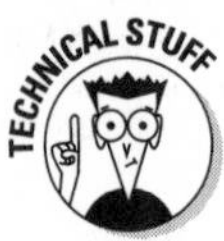

Osteoblasts (cells that build bone) make a protein known as *osteoprotegerin* (affectionately referred to as OPG). OPG binds to another protein, which activates osteoclasts. Therefore researchers have developed a compound that acts like OPG. They hope to turn this compound into a new drug that can increase bone density. *Phytoestrogens,* which are naturally occurring estrogens found in plants, may increase production of osteoprotegerin.

Again, much research will be needed before the general public might benefit from this information. For more information about new drugs on the horizon, see Chapter 10.

Repairing Collapsed Vertebrae: A New Surgical Treatment

One of the most devastating complications of osteoporosis is the bent back that results from collapsed vertebral bodies. The bent spine *(dowager's hump)* is due to *multiple compression fractures* (fracture of the vertebrae). To make matters worse, not only do these fractures cause deformities, but also they can cause severe and relentless pain.

A new surgical technique called *kyphoplasty* is a variation on a procedure known as vertebroplasty. (We describe vertebroplasty in Chapter 13.) *Kyphoplasty* is used in patients who have painful spinal fractures of less than one year's durations. Kyphoplasty uses an additional step in the vertebroplasty process that involves the use of a balloon to create a space inside the bone cavity so that more cement can be injected.

So essentially, a specialist (usually an orthopedist) inserts a large needle into the fractured bone, inflates a balloon, and injects acrylic cement, which hardens to keep the vertebrae in place.

Local anesthesia is used and some mild intravenous sedation. The initial results look promising with fewer complications compared to vertebroplasty.

No randomized clinical controlled trials have been conducted with this technique showing benefit of these procedures, but early results in more than 500 patients show promise. If you have collapsed vertebrae, consider this procedure only after obtaining several opinions. Make sure your surgeon has had a great deal of experience in performing this particular procedure.

Fighting Osteoporosis on an International Level

The effort to end osteoporosis is worldwide. Scientists are continually conducting research and attending seminars to discover ways to better prevent and treat osteoporosis. Two organizations have led the fight against osteoporosis worldwide:

- **The World Health Organization (WHO):** In the year 2000, WHO launched the "Bone and Joint Decade" 2000 to 2010 project. This international effort highlights the fact that public health officials have recognized the importance of musculoskeletal health. An international conference each year addresses topics including how to educate physicians and patients about osteoporosis and other problems affecting bones and joints. In 2004, 57 countries presented reports regarding their efforts to combat osteoporosis. For more information about the Bone and Joint Decade, click on `www.boneandjointdecade.org`.
- **The International Osteoporosis Foundation (IOF):** The IOF's mission is to improve early detection and treatment of osteoporosis by collaborating with national governments and healthcare systems throughout the world.

  The IOF has initiated many noteworthy and interesting programs, including the first Asia-wide campaign to alert women to the risk of developing osteoporosis. In October 2004, the organization ran a TV and print campaign in Asia urging women to take control of their bone health by taking the IOF "One Minute Osteoporosis Risk Test." In addition, the IOF showed three mannequins to graphically illustrate the three most common fractures due to osteoporosis (wrist, spine, and hip).

Part of the campaign also focuses on physicians and how they can do a better job of diagnosing and treating patients with osteoporosis.

The IOF (`www.osteofound.org`) also sponsors the International Congress on Osteoporosis, an annual meeting for health professionals to share the latest findings in bone health, and World Osteoporosis Day, an event that focuses each year on one particular issue related to osteoporosis. In 2004, the attention was on men.

Battling Osteoporosis in the United States

Organizations in the United States are also doing their share to end osteoporosis through education and prevention. The following represent just a few of the organizations working to battle osteoporosis in the United States.

- **The Surgeon General's Office:** While we were writing this book, the Surgeon General published a comprehensive report on osteoporosis. The document is 404 pages long (yes, it's a lot to read!) and demonstrates the interest that the United States Department of Health and Human Services has in improving bone health. The publication is free, and is available online, in print, and in CD format. It has everything a healthcare professional should know about osteoporosis and has great information for laymen as well. You can find the report at `www.http://www.surgeongeneral.gov/library/bonehealth/content.html`.
- **The National Committee for Quality Assurance:** This is a nonprofit oversight organization interested in assessing and improving performance of healthcare agencies in the United States. In 2004, the committee began to grade managed Medicare programs on their management of women who have suffered a fracture.
- **The National Institutes of Health (NIH):** The NIH has a wonderful program for educating the public about milk called "Milk Matters." The Web site (`www.nichd.nih.gov/milk`) contains valuable information.

Certain states have begun programs specifically addressing osteoporosis. Just a few examples include the following:

- **Michigan's Osteoporosis Project:** This project is a statewide program designed to reduce the prevalence of osteoporosis and reduce the number of osteoporosis-related fractures.
- **New Jersey's Project Healthy Bones:** This program is a 24-week exercise and osteoporosis education curriculum that emphasizes exercise, osteoporosis prevention, and treatment strategies as well as home safety and falls prevention.
- **North Carolina's Osteoporosis Coalition:** This program promotes education and support for prevention, diagnosis, and treatment of osteoporosis so as to achieve a reduction in its prevalence, severity, and costly consequences.

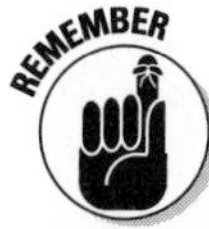

In addition, many states have started education programs aimed at children to stress the importance of diet and exercise in the development of strong bone. Some schools have gone so far as to remove soda vending machines from their buildings, replacing soft drinks with milk and juice. For much more about state legislation and to find out what your state is doing in the fight against osteoporosis, check out the Appendix.

Ongoing Research Regarding Osteoporosis

With new medications, education starting in childhood, and better detection methods, osteoporosis could, in the very near future, become a disease of the past. Education is one of the keys to changing the face of osteoporosis, and it needs to start — well, if not in kindergarten, then not long after.

Everyone needs to know that osteoporosis isn't a disease only of older women. (It can affect young people and men too.) And everyone needs to know that the habits you form and things you eat have lifelong effects on your bones.

What can you do if you already have osteoporosis? You can take advantage of today's technology and work on educating the next generation so that they'll never have to utilize it. Then we hope that one day in the not too distant future, your grandchildren will scratch their heads and ask, "Osteoporosis? What's that?"

Part IV
The Part of Tens

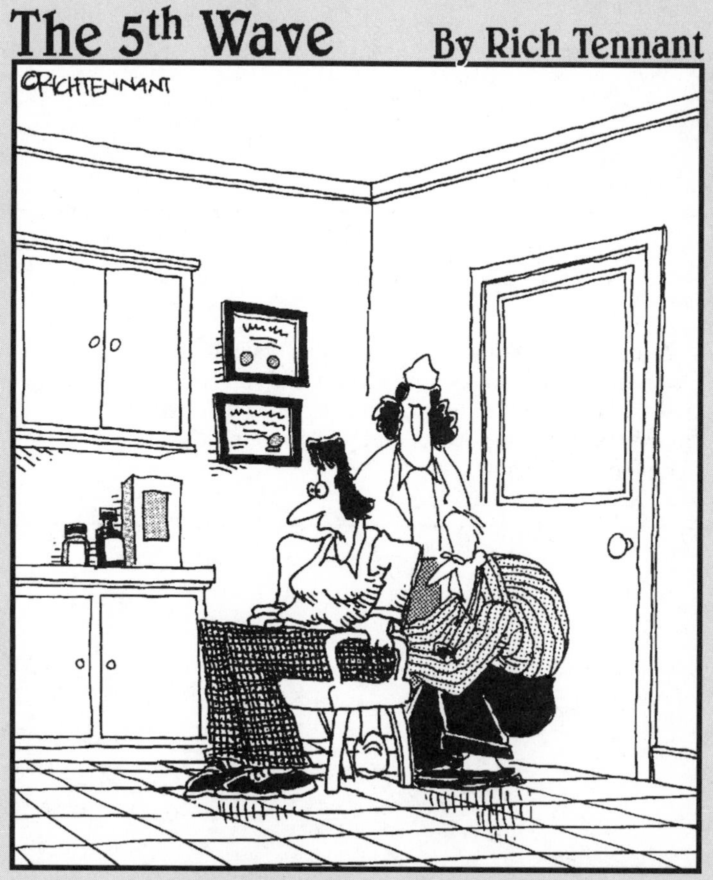

"I don't think the crackling sound coming from your lower back is as serious as you thought. Just relax and I'll have this Rice Krispie Square out of your back pocket in no time."

In this part . . .

Looking for some quick-and-easy ways to up your calcium intake? Want to know the top ten questions people ask about osteoporosis? Want to discover even more about osteoporosis and your bones? It's all here in The Part of Tens.

Chapter 15

Ten Surprising Sources of Calcium

In This Chapter

- Finding calcium in unusual places
- Trying mineral water
- Enjoying some high calcium dinners

If a glass of milk isn't exactly your cup of tea, you may think you're doomed to a calcium-deficient life. Don't despair — you can get your calcium from other sources outside the traditional milk carton.

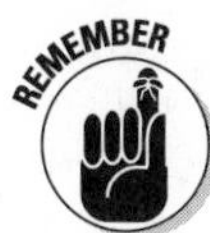

To help build strong bones that will carry you into your golden years, you need more than 1,000 mg of calcium each day, depending on your age (see Chapter 5 for more about daily calcium requirements by age). If your golden years are coming up quickly — that is, if you're older than 50 — you need at least 1,200 mg of calcium a day. That's almost as much as you need during your teen years (1,300 mg), when the foundation of your adult bone is being built.

In this chapter, we tell you how to fill your calcium requirements from sources you probably never thought of as good sources of calcium.

Drinking Mineral Water

Do you enjoy drinking mineral water but find it hard to justify the cost? It may help to know that a bottle of mineral water can contain anywhere from 25 to 400 mg of calcium per liter. Carrying a bottle of mineral water around with you is a great way to satisfy both your water and calcium requirements. Check labels to make sure you're getting the maximum amount of calcium for your dollars. To help you out, we include a few brands (and their country of origin) that have a high calcium level:

- Badoit (France): 190 mg per liter
- Borsec (Romania): 310 mg per liter
- Evian (France): 78 mg per liter
- Perrier (France): 147.3 mg per liter
- San Pellegrino (Italy): 208 mg per liter
- Vittel (France): 91 mg per liter

Going Beyond Leafy Green Veggies

Do you plug your nose at the smell of fresh green vegetables, such as spinach, broccoli, or romaine lettuce? Don't worry. If you don't like eating leafy greens, you can still hit the veggie tray and get your calcium from other vegetables.

Carrots contain 33 mg of calcium per cup, and cauliflower adds 22 mg per cup. Celery strips, which often seem like they're not valuable for anything except holding cream cheese or peanut butter, are good for 50 mg of calcium per cup. Add two tablespoons of cream cheese (25 mg) and you have 75 mg of calcium. (You can even eat healthier with fat-free or low-fat cream cheese and still get the same amount of calcium.) Eat a dozen, and you're almost up to your daily requirement!

Snap beans, green or yellow, add 41 mg per cup to your daily count, and if you're in the mood for Chinese, Chinese cabbage adds 74 mg per cup.

A cup of canned pumpkin is worth 64 mg of calcium. Mixed with a half cup of evaporated milk (350 mg) and poured into a small pastry shell, you've got pumpkin pie — and more than 400 mg of calcium in a single sitting. (We won't discuss the calorie count, however!)

Munching on Nuts and Seeds

Okay, so vegetables may not thrill you a whole lot more than milk does — how about some ideas for calcium that are more like treats and less like a chore to consume?

How about half a cup of almonds? How much easier could 200 mg of calcium be to ingest? You don't like almonds? How about pistachios (140 mg), macadamias (40 mg), or pecans (73 mg)?

Are you against nuts because they contain a lot of a fat and calories or are you allergic to nuts? How about sunflower seeds (140 mg)? Or sesame seeds (131 mg) ground into a wonderful sweet snack called halvah? Who said getting your calcium wasn't fun?

Eating Tacos for Dinner

Warm up the taco shells. Taco shells have 132 mg of calcium in one serving! Add the cheese (350 mg per serving), the sour cream (60 mg per ounce), and a plate of nachos with cheese (272 mg) before dinner and you've satisfied more than half your daily requirement and had a great time!

Sending Out for Pizza

Do you feel like staying home tonight and having a pizza delivered? One slice of cheese pizza contains 300 mg of calcium — and do you ever eat just one slice?

Taking One Latte to Go!

You may not like milk — but how about a latte? For some reason, it doesn't really taste like milk, does it? And one 12-ounce latte is good for 400 mg of calcium. If you don't want the caffeine buzz, you can always get a decaf.

Chugging a Little OJ Today

Can't start the morning without a glass of orange juice? Go ahead; one cup of fortified OJ contains 350 mg of calcium. Or try a different kind of snack. Nibbling on a bowlful of calcium-fortified cereal (without the milk) brings your breakfast total up to 500 mg to start the day. Or have a carton of low-fat yogurt (300 mg of calcium) for 650 mg of calcium to start your day.

Adding a Little Molasses

Are you looking for a sweetener that may actually have some health benefit? Try a little molasses. Two ounces contain 115 mg of calcium. You can find molasses in gingerbread and baked beans, if you don't feel like putting it on ice cream or eating it off the spoon.

Indulging on Chocolate Cake

One devil's food chocolate cake contains 1,100 mg of calcium. We're not advocating substituting the cake for a good day's intake of more healthy calcium-rich food, but isn't it nice to know that chocolate cake is good for something?

Powdering with a Different Twist

Do you ever think about nonfat powdered milk? A tablespoon of nonfat powdered milk contains 52 mg of calcium, and you can toss a few tablespoons into everything from gravy to homemade cookies. Keep a box handy and increase your calcium intake without even noticing it!

Chapter 16

Ten Things You Need to Know about Bones

In This Chapter

- Counting up the benefits of having healthy bones
- Making healthy bones a lifelong priority
- Finding reasons to keep your bones together

Having healthy bones and avoiding osteoporosis has, for many of you, become just one more health chore that you know you need to do, but you just may have not gotten around to it. Your co-author Sharon's sister, an X-ray tech who works for a group of orthopedic doctors, said, "Bones are so boring" when Sharon first talked about writing this book. Undoubtedly, many of you can relate and agree with Sharon's sister.

Okay, so bones are boring. Talking about taking your calcium and eating your vegetables can be dull. Even though thinking about bones may be boring, taking care of them isn't boring if you realize how important they are. In this chapter, we give you ten very interesting reasons why you need to pay attention to your bones throughout your lifetime.

Broken Bones Hurt!

If you've ever had one, you know having a broken bone hurts. And if you've been fortunate and never had one, just ask someone who has and she'll tell you all about the pain.

Not only do broken bones hurt, but they also take a long time to heal. If you break an arm or leg, you may spend six weeks in a cast. If you break a hip, you'll be on crutches for months. For a graphic illustration, borrow a pair of crutches and see how much fun it is to use them in the bathroom.

Or, for even more graphic fun, wrap some type of bandage around your arm for a day and then imagine it there for several weeks. Your skin gets all flaky under the cast, and it gets really itchy, too. You go crazy trying to think of ways to scratch through the cast. And when you take the cast off, your arm is skinny and gray — not to mention flaky.

Broken Bones Can Make You Sick — or Worse

The mortality rate from broken bones, especially hips, is very high. The fracture itself may not cause further illness, but the inability to move around can. In fact, a rather frightening 24 percent of hip fracture patients older than age 50 die within one year of their fracture. Two-thirds of those who fracture a bone never fully recover their former quality of life.

If you're in bed for a long time, you're more likely to develop blood clots or pneumonia, illnesses that can lead to the most serious consequence of broken bones — death within the year of a fracture.

Having a broken hip can lead to permanent residence in a nursing home. One quarter of those who were able to walk unaided before their fracture ended up needing permanent nursing care after their fracture.

Increasing Calcium Certainly Helps Decrease Fractures

Some research suggests that as many as 40 to 60 percent of osteoporotic-related hip fractures could have been avoided if people would just consume enough calcium. We give you some great and painless ways to take in your recommended daily amount of calcium in Chapter 15. The older you get, the more calcium you need.

Milk Is Really Important to Bone

One cup of milk provides one-fourth of your daily requirement of calcium and one-fourth of your daily requirement of vitamin D, both of which are important for bone growth and health (see Chapter 5 for more about diet).

The power of milk to increase your daily calcium intake is why your parents probably taught you to drink four glasses of milk each day.

You Don't Get a Second Chance at Building Bone

Don't wait until you're 70 before you start thinking about your bones. You actually finish building bones by your 30s; after that, you can replace what's lost, but you can't increase what you have.

This news doesn't mean you can't still improve your bone strength at age 70. In fact, you can help keep what you have by eating well, exercising, and avoiding excess alcohol and smoking. But you can't increase the bone you have at this point. The bone you built before your 30s is all you're ever going to have.

Today's Bad Habits Lead to Tomorrow's Bone Loss

In some areas of life, you can put your bad habits aside after you reach your 30s and 40s and live as though you never made them. But when it comes to your bones, yesterday's bad habits affect the amount of bone you have for the rest of you life!

Lack of exercise, smoking, and drinking too much alcohol will catch up to you later in life. Losing bone density is only one of the consequences of bad habits, but it's an important one.

Develop an exercise program with your doctor, stop drinking excessively, and throw away your cigarettes. (If you need help with the latter, check out *Quitting Smoking For Dummies* by David Brizer, MD, [Wiley].) Make sure you're passing these bits of wisdom on to the next generations; they'll thank you in the future.

Getting Shorter Is No Fun at All

If osteoporosis added inches instead of subtracting them, it might not be such a bad thing. But because many people go through life wishing to be a little taller, the prospect of losing what little height they have isn't a pleasant one!

Growing shorter may be a problem on your wallet because you have to spend more money buying clothes that fit. However, the loss of height caused by fractured vertebrae is more costly to your health because it can also cause the following (to name a few of the more serious side effects):

- It makes deep breathing difficult.
- It decreases your appetite because your stomach feels squashed.
- It results in weight loss that you may not be able to afford.

Your Bones Are a Storehouse of Necessary Minerals

Bones do more than help you stand up; they're also the storehouses of a large amount of the minerals you need to keep every system in your body functioning. Your bones store 99 percent of your body's calcium, along with 85 percent of phosphorus, 60 percent of magnesium, and 35 percent of sodium. These minerals give strength and rigidity to our bones, and serve as a reservoir of minerals that the rest of your body can draw on to keep every system in your body functioning properly.

Broken Bones Cost Society a Ton of Money

You may not be that concerned about costing society money. But the fact is that society's money is really everyone's money, so money lost by hospitals, workplaces, and the government eventually costs everyone, including yourself, in higher prices and taxes.

A 1996 report by the National Osteoporosis Foundation (NOF) reported that the cost of treating osteoporotic fractures was between $13 and $18 billion (yes, *billion!*) a year. That study is nearly ten years old so the costs have probably risen. Rehabilitation and institutionalization accounted for about 40 percent, and inpatient hospital care about 25 percent of the cost. The cost of premature death accounted for another 33 percent, with 1 percent or so due to lost time in the workplace.

These costs are only going to rise as the population ages and as more people age 65 and above fall down and break something.

Bones Turn Over All the Time

Eating well and exercising for a week or two isn't enough to maintain strong bone, because bone is being broken down and rebuilt all the time. You have to make eating well and exercising a part of your everyday life.

Before you turned a year old, nearly 100 percent of your bone had been replaced by new bone. As an adult, about 10 percent of your bone is replaced each year.

Bone remodeling is a 24-hour a day operation; old bone is constantly being removed and new bone being laid down. Anything that disrupts the process of new bone building, such as a lack of calcium or vitamin D, affects the amount and type of new bone growth.

Chapter 17

Ten Resources for Finding Out More about Osteoporosis

In This Chapter

- Uncovering more info about osteoporosis
- Trying a support group
- Perusing books and Web sites
- Discussing osteoporosis with your doctor

You may want to know more about osteoporosis than we can tell you in this book. The good news is that plenty of information is available for you out there. You just have to uncover it.

In this chapter, we tell you how to find the latest updates, the newest studies, the most supportive support groups, and other resources to keep you in the know about what's going on with osteoporosis.

Staying Up-to-Date with the NOF

Started in 1984, the National Osteoporosis Foundation (NOF) promotes awareness, public and professional education, advocacy, and research. The NOF is a nonprofit organization; membership is currently $15 per year within the United States.

Membership buys you a quarterly newsletter called *Osteoporosis Report* and a 70-page booklet called *Boning Up On Osteoporosis.* The Web site (`www.nof.org`) also includes a list of doctors specializing in osteoporosis treatment. Keep in mind that the doctors listed pay to be listed, and aren't endorsed by the NOF.

The NOF also helps set up support groups for osteoporosis called *Building Strength Together* around the country. (See the "Joining a

Support Group" section in this chapter for more information on how it works.)

The NOF also sells books, exercise tapes, and promotional material related to osteoporosis on its Web site. If you're not comfortable surfing the Internet, you can contact the organization to request materials at

National Osteoporosis Foundation

1232 22nd St. N.W.

Washington, DC 20037

202-223-2226

Relying on the NIH

The National Institutes of Health (NIH) is associated with two sources of information on osteoporosis: the National Institute of Aging Information Center and the NIH Osteoporosis and Related Bone Disease-National Resource Center.

- The first resource is a branch of the NIH called the **National Institute on Aging Information Center (NIAIC).** NIAIC's Web site (www.nih.gov/nia) is a wealth of information on clinical trials and research, not only related to osteoporosis, but also about aging in general. You can order publications on a number of topics related to osteoporosis and aging.

  You can reach the NIAIC in a number of ways. You can e-mail at niaic@jbsl.com, or call at 800-222-2225 or 800-222-4225 (TTY). If you want to send away for information, write

  NIAIC

  P.O. Box 8057

  Gaithersburg, MD 20898

- The second resource is associated with the **NIH Osteoporosis and Related Bone Diseases-National Resource Center.** The organization's Web site (www.osteo.org) has many fact sheets that you can download or have mailed to you.

  If you want to snail mail the organization, write to

  NIH ORBD-NRC

  2 AMS Circle

  Bethesda, MD 20892

  Or call 800-624-BONE

Utilizing Expert Medical Facilities

Harvard Medical School and the Mayo Clinic are two well known medical facilities that publish a plethora of medical information of just about any topic you can name, including osteoporosis, exercise, and diet.

Harvard publishes a number of 30- to 50-page pamphlets on topics such as *Boosting Bone Strength* for $16 each. (Prices may be subject to change.) In addition, the Web site (`www.health.harvard.edu/newsletters/special.html`) contains a copious number of articles and information on osteoporosis and related subjects. You also can call Harvard Health publications at 877-649-9457 or e-mail them at `harvardpro@palmcoastd.com`.

The Mayo Clinic is well known as a prolific publisher of health information for consumers as well. Mayo's Web site (`www.mayoclinic.com`) is a wealth of information on many health issues; you can also subscribe to a free newsletter.

Joining a Support Group

Talking and commiserating with a group of people who know what you're going through because they've also gone through the same situation can help you deal with your condition. Support groups are everywhere, and you can find osteoporosis support groups in most large cities and quite a few small ones as well.

The NOF (see the "Staying Up-to-Date with the NOF" section earlier in this chapter) sponsors and helps set up support groups around the country under the name *Building Strength Together (BST)*. The NOF supplies materials, referrals, a manual to help you know where to start, and technical support. If you go to the NOF's Web site (`www.nof.org`), you can find a link to applications to join support groups separated by age and gender.

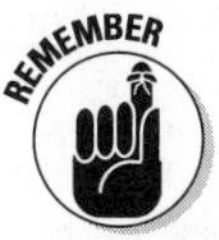

Your local newspaper may have a section that lists area meetings. You can also utilize your nearest hospital; many groups meet at or are sponsored by area hospitals.

Chatting Online about Osteoporosis

No matter what subject interests you, you can be assured that someone else out there is also interested and wants someone to talk to about it on the Internet.

Osteoporosis is no exception. Nearly all the large Internet providers, such as Yahoo!, AOL, and MSN, sponsor support groups for every disease known to man, including osteoporosis. Just type "osteoporosis support" into your search bar and click on the results.

Some groups are far more active than others by holding local meetings among people who live near each other. If your first encounter turns out to be a dud, don't despair — plenty of groups are out there! You may find some people who chat in more than one group — and you can do the same!

The great thing about online bulletin boards and chatrooms is that they never close. When you wake up at 4 a.m. and can't sleep, you can log in and talk to another insomniac. You can also remain anonymous if you want, and can ask questions that you may not feel comfortable asking your best friends!

Just remember that the people you're chatting with aren't experts and may have outdated or just plain wrong information! You don't know exactly who you're talking to, so if you have any questions about what someone says in a chatroom, consult your doctor. One problem with the Internet is that people can easily sound like an "expert" when they're not, or to pretend to be someone — like a nurse or a physician — when they're not.

Reading Books

If you're a reader, you're in luck! Although we obviously think this book is a great resource for osteoporosis, many other books on osteoporosis are available. In addition, books, such as *Fitness Over 40 For Dummies* by Betsy Nagelsen McCormack and Mike Yorkey and *Weight Training For Dummies,* 2nd Edition, by Liz Neporent and Suzanne Schlosberg (both by Wiley), can help you put your newfound intentions to exercise your way to better bones to good use.

Watching Videos

Are you not the type who likes to read books (except this book, of course)? You can choose from numerous videotapes, such as *Exercise: A Video from the National Institute on Aging*, a 48-minute video. It comes with a companion booklet. You can find more information at www.niapublications.org/exercisevideo/index.asp.

Talking with Your Doctor about Osteoporosis

Don't overlook your doctor as a source of up-to-date information on the latest drugs and studies related to osteoporosis. Most doctors receive at least one journal a month filled with the latest medical advances.

Although most doctors aren't willing to have you call them up just to chat about what's new in osteoporosis, they often will call you back if you have specific questions about something you've seen or read about.

Visiting Your Favorite Physical Therapist

Physical therapists are important health professionals with master's degrees who are specially trained to give you an individualized exercise program that strengthens your bones. They conduct a complete evaluation to understand exactly what your needs are, determine if you have any weak areas that need to be protected, and design a program just for you. Then they monitor your progress and determine if the exercises need to be changed. Usually your primary care doctor, rheumatologist, or orthopedic surgeon will know the most qualified physical therapists in your area.

For additional information, contact the Association of Rheumatology Health Professionals, 1800 Century Place, Suite 250, Atlanta, GA 30345; phone 404-633-3777.

Going Online for the Latest Information

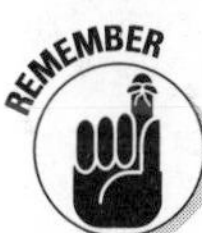

The Internet is a wonderful source of information, but keep in mind that some of the information may be rumor, wishful thinking, or just plain out-to-lunch thinking. Just remember that with the Internet, everyone can play — and some Web sites contain incorrect or inflammatory information that they pass off as the hidden — usually "government-suppressed" — truth.

To find more information on osteoporosis than you could read in a year, just go to your favorite search engine and type in "osteoporosis." Approximately 4 million sites will appear, although in all honesty, many of them are duplicates of the same information. You'll still have plenty of reading material to keep you busy for a long, long time. Drug companies developing medications that prevent and treat osteoporosis often have educational material that is available on the Web. (Okay, so these sites aren't exactly an unbiased source of information, because the drug companies are naturally promoting their own drugs, but these sites are still a valuable resource on the available drugs.)

Check out the following Web sites if you're itching for more information on osteoporosis.

- `www.medscape.com` and `www.medlineplus.com` provide some of the latest articles on osteoporosis published in medical journals.
- Merck's `www.fosamax.com`, Procter & Gamble Pharmaceutical's site `www.fightfractures.com`, and Eli Lilly's `www.forteo.com` offer information about these three drug company's specific osteoporosis drugs.
- `www.rheumatology.org/public/factsheets` is the Web site for the American College of Rheumatology, the professional organization of rheumatologists. (*Rheumatologists* are qualified by additional training and experience in the diagnosis and treatment of arthritis and other diseases of the joints, muscles, and bones.) The site has information sheets regarding osteoporosis and corticosteroids-related osteoporosis. You can also use this site to locate a rheumatologist in your neighborhood. One physician who is an expert on osteoporosis has a great Web site at `http://faculty.washington.edu/smott/`.
- `www.surgeongeneral.gov/library/bonehealth/content.html` is where you can check out the Surgeon General's Report on the latest official word on osteoporosis. It contains up-to-date and complete downloadable information — 437 pages worth.
- `www.gotmilk.com` or `//www.whymilk.com/` provides a lighter glance. The International Dairy Foods has sponsored the Got Milk? campaign, which celebrated its tenth year in 2003. Its catchy slogans and billboard ads have raised awareness of the importance of milk in the development of healthy bones. See these sites for the latest and greatest about milk and bones.
- `http://vitamind.ucr.edu/about.html` is a site run by a society that sponsors research about vitamin D. The site describes everything you need to know about vitamin D.

Chapter 18

Top Ten Questions Dr. O'Connor's Patients Ask about Osteoporosis

In This Chapter

- Figuring out what real people really want to know about osteoporosis
- Finding out what you need to know

No question is too silly or unimportant to ask. In this chapter, Dr. O'Connor answers the questions she hears most commonly. We suspect that you may have thought of the same questions at one time or another. We also include a chapter reference for you if you want more than just the short answer!

What's the Best Type of Calcium for Me?

Answer: The cheapest!

Seriously, the most easily absorbed form of calcium is calcium citrate, but the most important consideration about calcium intake is to take enough. Don't worry so much about the type of calcium. Instead, find the least expensive kind. (See Chapter 11 for more on calcium supplements.)

How Much Calcium Do I Need Each Day?

Answer: It varies with your age.

Because your ability to absorb calcium decreases with age, you need more calcium when you're older than 55. I generally recommend 1,500 mg daily for that age group. (See Chapter 5 for more info on different age groups.)

I Drink Plenty of Milk. Isn't That Enough Calcium for My Bones?

Answer: Yes, but only if you really do drink *a lot* of milk.

One cup of unfortified milk supplies 300 mg of calcium. Therefore you need at least four cups of milk every day if you're older than 55. Drinking milk is a fabulous way to get calcium in your diet. Calcium from food is more easily absorbed than calcium from supplementation. (See Chapters 5 and 11 for more on calcium.)

What Exercises Are Best for Preventing Osteoporosis?

Answer: The general rule is 30 minutes of weight-bearing exercise (such as walking and stair climbing) daily. See Chapter 6 for a more complete exercise program.

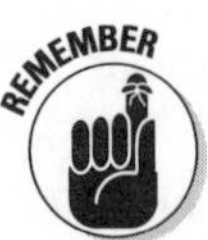

Before you start any exercise program, consult your physician.

What's the Difference between Osteoporosis and Osteoarthritis?

Answer: They're completely different problems.

Osteoporosis is the most common cause of fragile *bones,* while osteoarthritis is a problem with your *joints* (such as your knees or hips). Osteoarthritis causes pain in your joints at an early stage, whereas osteoporosis is painless at an early stage. (See Chapter 1 for more on osteoarthritis.)

My Back Hurts. Is That My Osteoporosis?

Answer: No, fragile, osteoporotic bones don't hurt!

The only time you'll have pain with osteoporosis is after a fracture. (See Chapters 7 and 13 for more on vertebral compression fractures.) If your back hurts, don't blame it on your low bone density. See your physician!

What Else Can I Do to Improve Bone Strength?

Answer: Stop smoking, limit alcohol intake, and make sure that you have a minimum of 800 International Units (IU) of vitamin D daily. (See Chapter 3 for more on risk factors for osteoporosis.)

My Family Doc Recommended a Bone Density Study. How Is It Done?

Answer: No preparation is necessary other than not taking your calcium tablets for 24 hours prior to the test. The density of your left hip and lower spine are measured with a specialized X-ray. There is no injection or pain. This simple test takes 15 or 20 minutes, and the amount of radiation received is less than what you would get from a standard chest X-ray.

(See Chapter 9 for more on testing your bone density.)

Which Is Better, Alendronate or Risedronate?

Answer: Research has shown that both prevent osteoporotic fractures.

To my knowledge, no head-to-head studies have compared these drugs with each other. (See Chapter 10 for more on different osteoporosis medications.)

I've Had a Curved Spine Since My Teenage Years. Do I Have Osteoporosis?

Answer: Probably not.

When your parents insisted that you weren't standing up straight, you may have had a curvature of your spine known as *scoliosis.* This condition has nothing to do with osteoporosis, other than the fact that both scoliosis and osteoporosis cause loss of height. (See Chapter 1 for more on differentiation between these two diseases.)

Chapter 19

Ten (Or So) Parenting Tips to Build Strong Bones

In This Chapter

- Preventing osteoporosis in the next generation
- Instilling healthy habits in your children (and grandchildren)

Most parents (and grandparents) want to do everything they can to ensure their children (and grandchildren) grow up healthy and lead long lives. That includes helping them develop strong bones. (You do want Little Emma and Ethan to grow up big and strong, right?) Remember that bone health in adults depends upon critical factors in childhood.

In this chapter, we give you ten (or so) things you need to know as a parent (and as a grandparent) to lower your children's (and grandchildren's) risk of developing osteoporosis.

The More You Exercise, the Stronger Your Bones Will Be

Children need to be active starting from toddler ages to teenage years. Don't let your kids (and grandkids) become couch potatoes or computer addicts! The more weight-bearing activity, such as running and walking, that they do during the growing years, the better their bones will be later.

Better yet, get out there and play a game of softball or Frisbee or take a bike ride with them, and the entire family will have healthier bones. (Check out Chapter 6 for more information on exercise.)

Drinking Milk Daily Builds Big Benefits for Bones

Just four glasses of milk each day — one with each meal and one for a snack — gives you enough calcium and vitamin D for your bones to develop properly. Calcium requirements increase during adolescence and teenage years, at the very ages when kids may be least likely to eat well and drink enough milk.

The daily requirement for calcium at age 9 to 18 is 1,300 mg a day. Check out Chapter 5 for ways to increase calcium intake painlessly, and Chapter 15 for some great ways to get calcium if your child is allergic to milk.

Shopping Wisely Is Worth the Extra Time

When you shop for your family, read food labels to check for the calcium and vitamin D content in the foods you buy. The extra time it takes to check for calcium and vitamin D can pay off in better bones for you all. For example, soymilk now states, "fortified" on the carton, which means that vitamin D has been added.

Don't Let Lactose Intolerance Rob Your Child of Calcium

Does your child (or grandchild) suffer from lactose intolerance? Lactose intolerance means that they can't break down and use *lactose,* the main sugar found in milk and other dairy products. The symptoms include bloating, lower abdominal pains, and loose stools after drinking milk. As time goes by, people who are lactose intolerant often drink less milk to avoid the symptoms, which is definitely not what you want for your child.

Dr. O'Connor had a small victory while she was working on this book. Her son, who is lactose intolerant, was home from college. She was working on the chapter about nutrition, and she encouraged him to read labels for the calcium and vitamin D amounts. That evening for dinner he had a large glass of soymilk. Better yet, she reports that her house now doesn't have any soft drinks. (See the next section for more info on soft drinks.)

If your child can't drink milk because of lactose intolerance, then supplement with calcium tablets or soymilk. Check out Chapter 5 for ideas on ways to maintain an adequate calcium intake if your child (or grandchild) is lactose intolerant.

Avoid Carbonated Beverages

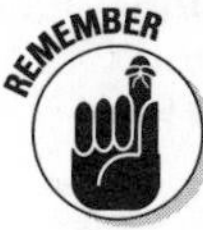

Although an occasional soft drink is fine, don't let soda take the place of milk in your children's diet. Carbonated drinks contain phosphoric acid, which can cause calcium loss in your child's bones. A better alternative is to replace the soft drinks with milk and calcium-fortified juices.

Watch for Signs of Anorexia

If your child (or grandchild) is severely underweight, you need to keep an eye open for the warning signals of anorexia nervosa. Anorexia is a serious psychiatric disorder where people have a distorted body image and where they're intensely afraid to gain weight or become fat, even though they're underweight.

Also keep your eyes open in case your teenage daughter (or granddaughter) has erratic menstrual cycles. If you notice any of these symptoms, consult your physician as soon as possible, before the problem has time to become more serious. (See Chapter 4 for more about anorexia nervosa.)

When someone is anorexic, they're typically not eating well or taking in the necessary calcium and vitamin D. As a result, the condition has long-term consequences on bone health.

Know Your Family History

Heredity is extremely important in understanding one's risk for developing osteoporosis. Let your children (and grandchildren) know if someone in your family has osteoporosis so that they can carry that information with them into the future.

If your children (or grandchildren) know that their great-grandma on mom's side and their dad's mom each suffered from osteoporosis, they may think again before they skip their daily calcium intake. Then again, you may have to remind them.

Set an Example about Eating Healthy

Yes, children watch and emulate their parents and even their grandparents, even though at times it seems that they do the exact opposite! Little eyes are watching — if your breakfast consists of coffee and a donut, what will your children consider good nutrition as they grow up? Make a decision to include calcium-rich and vitamin D–fortified foods to all your meals. (For instance, skip the donut and eat a cup of yogurt.)

How much better — for all of you — if your diet choices show that eating well is important to you. Children really do pay more attention to what parents do than to what they say!

Help Your Teen Avoid Cigarettes and Alcohol

Talking to your kids about the risks of smoking and drinking is an important way to prevent your children from picking up either as a bad habit. Smoking and drinking not only have detrimental effects on your bone health, but on so many other parts of your body. (And don't forget that smoking is an expensive, dirty habit.)

Although peer pressure is strong, parents really do have an equally strong influence on their kids. Make sure your offspring know where you stand — and of course, set the proper example.

Appendix

Reviewing Osteoporosis Programs State by State

In This Appendix

- Checking out your state's osteoporosis legislation
- Finding state programs that may benefit you

As you may remember from history, states don't always see eye to eye. This statement is evident when you check out each of the 50 states and their laws and programs related to osteoporosis. Some have great insurance coverage and wonderful educational programs, while some have nothing.

In this appendix, we give you a state-by-state review so you can see how your state stacks up to others about putting the spotlight on osteoporosis. If your state has no programs for osteoporosis detection or prevention, call your representative and ask why!

Alabama

In 1995, Alabama created the *Osteoporosis Prevention and Treatment Education Act* to increase public awareness of osteoporosis and educate the public about the causes, risk factors, prevention, and treatment options. Check out `www.adph.org/NUTRITION/default.asp?DeptId=115&TemplateId=2022& TemplateNbr=0` for more information.

Alaska

Alaska has a combined program called the Alaska Arthritis and Osteoporosis Plan that works to educate the public on both diseases through education, mentoring, and care to remote underserved areas. The Web site is `www.epi.hss.state.ak.us`.

Arizona

The Arizona Osteoporosis Coalition strives to raise awareness of osteoporosis through education, communications, and public activity. The Web site is www.azoc.org/. The University of Arizona Cooperative Extension also spearheads a program called Bone Builders, an osteoporosis prevention education program targeting women and older men. Visit the Web site at www.bonebuilders.org/.

Arkansas

The *Osteoporosis Prevention and Treatment Act* was passed in 1997 in Arkansas, and requires the health department to coordinate with other agencies and organizations to establish, promote, and maintain an osteoporosis program geared toward prevention and treatment education. The program's purpose is to raise public awareness, educate consumers, and educate and train health professionals and service providers. The University of Arkansas also has a Web site packed with information on osteoporosis; go to www.arfamilies.org/health/Osteoporosis_and_Arthritis.

California

California is one of the few states to require insurance companies to provide coverage for the diagnosis, treatment, and appropriate management of osteoporosis. This coverage includes all technologies approved by the Federal Drug Administration (FDA) and bone mass measurement technologies as deemed medically appropriate.

In addition, The California Osteoporosis Prevention and Education (COPE) program, established in 1999, promotes, develops, and implements public health interventions for the prevention of osteoporosis and osteoporosis-related disability for all Californians aged 50 and older. California's Web site for osteoporosis is www.dhs.ca.gov/osteoporosis. California also has a program aimed at reaching low-income Latino mothers. You can find more information at www.californiaprojectlean.org/programs/bonehealth.

Colorado

Colorado has no current legislation, but you can find information at www.cdphe.state.co.us/pp/osteoporosis/osteohom.html.

Connecticut

Connecticut has had an advisory council on osteoporosis and a task force to study the availability of resources to treat and diagnose osteoporosis in the past; both have expired. Connecticut also has an education program directed at children through Head Start, using a character called "Captain 5 A Day" to educate youngsters about good nutrition. Check out the Captain's Web site at www.dph.state.ct.us/BCH/HEI/Captain5ADayWebsite.htm.

Delaware

In 1998, Delaware established the Osteoporosis Prevention and Education Initiative within the Department of Health and Social Services to promote and maintain an osteoporosis prevention and education initiative. The initiative's goal is to raise public awareness of the causes and nature of osteoporosis, personal risk factors, and the value of prevention and early detection. (Check out www.delaware.gov/ and type "osteoporosis" in the search engine for many details.)

District of Columbia

No current legislation exists.

Florida

Florida, home to many retired men and women, requires insurers to provide coverage for medically necessary diagnosis and treatment of osteoporosis for high-risk individuals, with some exceptions.

In 1996, Florida created the Osteoporosis Prevention and Education Program to promote public awareness of the causes of osteoporosis, options for prevention, the value of early detection, and possible treatments, including the benefits and risks of those treatments. Florida also maintains a Web site for osteoporosis: www.doh.state.fl.us/family/osteo.

Georgia

Georgia's *Bone Mass Measurement Coverage Act,* passed in 1998, requires insurance plans to offer coverage for scientifically proven bone mass measurement for the prevention, diagnosis, and treatment of osteoporosis.

Since 1995, Georgia's *Osteoporosis Prevention and Treatment Education Act* offers a multigenerational, statewide program to promote awareness and knowledge about osteoporosis, risk factors, prevention, detection, and treatment options. Georgia's osteoporosis Web site is `www.gabones.com`.

Hawaii

No current legislation exists.

Idaho

No current legislation exists.

Illinois

The Illinois Department of Public Health was charged in 1996 with establishing, promoting, and maintaining an osteoporosis prevention and education program to promote public awareness of the causes of osteoporosis. In addition, in 2001 the *Senior Citizens and Disabled Persons Property Tax Relief and Pharmaceutical Assistance Act* required added coverage for any prescription drug used in the treatment of osteoporosis. (Look at `www.idph.state.il.us/about/womenshealth/factsheets/osteo.htm` for more information.)

Indiana

The Indiana Department of Health established an osteoporosis prevention and treatment program and an education fund in 1997. The Web site is `www.in.gov/isdh/programs/osteo/index.htm`.

Iowa

No current legislation exists.

Kansas

In 2001, the legislature enacted a law that requires insurers to provide coverage for the diagnosis, treatment, and management of osteoporosis, including bone mineral density testing where medically necessary. (Click on `www.accesskansas.org/` and enter "osteoporosis" in the search engine for numerous resources.)

Kentucky

Legislation enacted in 1998 requires insurers to offer coverage for bone mineral density testing for women age 35 and older to obtain a baseline measurement for early detection of osteoporosis. The Web site is `http://chfs.ky.gov/`.

Louisiana

Legislation passed in 1999 requires insurers to include coverage for scientifically proven bone mass measurement for the diagnosis and treatment of osteoporosis.

Maine

No current legislation exists.

Maryland

Maryland established an Osteoporosis Prevention and Education Task Force in 2002. Maryland also requires coverage for reimbursement of bone mass measurement for individuals when a healthcare provider requests a measurement. `StrongerBones.org` is a Web site devoted to promoting bone health and preventing osteoporosis provided by the Maryland Department of Health and Mental Hygiene's Office of Chronic Disease Prevention.

Massachusetts

The Massachusetts Osteoporosis Awareness Program, started in 1993, encompasses residents from children to the elderly, men and women, and promotes prevention, screening, and treatment information at every age. The Web site is www.state.ma.us/dph/bfch/chp/nutphys/osteo.htm.

Michigan

In 1997 and 1998, the Michigan legislature allotted funds to be used for health education, research, prevention, and treatment programs for osteoporosis. The Web site is www.michigan.gov/osteoporosis. (To read more about this program, check out Chapter 14.)

Minnesota

An appropriations bill in 1995 required the Minnesota Department of Health to report on the need for an osteoporosis prevention and treatment program, and authorized the department to apply for grants and gifts to establish the program.

Mississippi

In 1994 Mississippi was ahead of most other states and established the *Osteoporosis Prevention and Treatment Education Act* to promote awareness and education about the causes, prevention, and treatment of osteoporosis. (Check out www.mississippi.gov/index.jsp and type "osteoporosis" in the search engine for details.)

Missouri

The Missouri Department of Health started promoting and maintaining an osteoporosis prevention and education program in 1995. This legislation also allowed the department to establish an osteoporosis advisory council. The Web site is www.dhss.mo.gov/maop.

Montana

No current legislation exists.

Nebraska

No current legislation exists.

Nevada

In Nevada, the week beginning with Mother's Day is Osteoporosis Prevention and Awareness Week. (What about the fathers who have osteoporosis? We were wondering the same thing.) Nevada also has initiated a campaign to increase calcium intake in 11- to 14-year-olds called "Calcium — It's Not Just Milk." The Web site for this program is `www.unce.unr.edu./nvfsnep` under Programs.

New Hampshire

In 1997, the New Hampshire Department of Health and Human Services started an osteoporosis awareness program to educate, prevent, and treat osteoporosis. You can find information on the state program at `www.gencourt.state.nh.us/rsa/html/indexes/126-I.html`.

New Jersey

In 1997, New Jersey established an osteoporosis prevention and education program through the Department of Health and Senior Services called New Jersey Interagency Council on Osteoporosis. Their vision is simple: to STOP osteoporosis — Screen, Treat, Overcome, Prevent. The program's Web site is `www.state.nj.us/health/senior/osteo`. (To read more about this program, refer to Chapter 14.)

New Jersey also reaches out to educate children with "KidStrong (Inside & Out)," an educational prevention program aimed at educating fifth and sixth graders, and "Jump Start Your Bones," a school-based osteoporosis prevention curriculum for seventh and eighth graders. You can view the curriculum at `www.njfsnep.org`.

New Mexico

Funds were allocated in 1998 for an osteoporosis prevention, treatment, and education program. (Link to www.state.nm.us/ and type "osteoporosis" in the search engine for more resources.)

New York

Since 1998, New York's Osteoporosis Prevention and Education Program has promoted public awareness of osteoporosis, including public education and an outreach campaign. In 2002, New York required that certain health insurance contracts provide coverage for bone mineral density testing, as well as FDA-approved prescription drugs. The Web site is http://nysopep.org.

North Carolina

Since 1999, North Carolina has required insurance companies to provide coverage for scientifically proven and approved bone mass measurement for the diagnosis and evaluation of osteoporosis. Prior to that, the Osteoporosis Task Force was created in 1997 to raise public awareness, obtain statistical data, and develop an osteoporosis prevention plan. (See www.communityhealth.dhhs.state.nc.us/oldadult.htm for more information.)

North Dakota

No current legislation exists.

Ohio

In 1997, funds were appropriated for the Osteoporosis Awareness Program in 1997. The program's Web site is www.odh.ohio.gov/odhprograms/sadv/womenhlth/costeo.pdf.

Oklahoma

In 1996, the state required insurers to provide coverage for bone mineral density testing to people at risk for osteoporosis, when a primary care or referral physician requests the testing.

Oklahoma also has an osteoporosis prevention, treatment, and education program within the Oklahoma Department of Health and the Interagency Council on Osteoporosis. Go to its Web site at www.health.state.ok.us and type in "osteoporosis" for more information.

Oregon

No current legislation exists.

Pennsylvania

The Pennsylvania Osteoporosis Strategic Plan, released in September 2004, intends to reduce the burden of osteoporosis by focusing on educating its citizens on the three ages and stages important to prevention of osteoporosis: the Bone Building Years (0 to 30), the Bone Maintenance Years (30 to 50), and the Bone Loss Years (50 and older). A risk assessment of the general population based on age, race, gender, and geographical areas can help reduce the impact of the disease on different stages of life, because evidence shows that education started in adolescence and continued throughout the different stages of life helps improve healthy outcomes.

The Pennsylvania Osteoporosis Prevention and Education Strategic Plan was a result of the collaboration between the Department of Health and the Pennsylvania Osteoporosis Coalition, and reflects the commitment to address the serious problems of osteoporosis and other chronic diseases. The Web site is www.dsf.health.state.pa.us/health/lib/health/Osteoporosis.pdf.

Rhode Island

Since 2001, Rhode Island has provided pharmaceutical assistance to the elderly for FDA-approved drugs used to treat osteoporosis. Rhode Island's Web site is www.health.ri.gov/disease/osteoporosis/index.htm.

South Carolina

The state legislature established the *Osteoporosis Prevention, Treatment, and Education Act* and an *Osteoporosis Education Fund* to promote public awareness and education. You can find more information on South Carolina's Department of Health Web site at www.scdhec.gov/health/hhealth/arthritis. Type "osteoporosis" into the search engine for a link to relevant articles.

South Dakota

No current legislation exists.

Tennessee

May is designated Osteoporosis Prevention Month in Tennessee. The state has required insurers to provide coverage for scientifically proven bone mass measurement since 1996 and created the *Osteoporosis Prevention and Treatment Education Act* in 1995. The state Web site is www.state.tn.us. Type "osteoporosis" into the search engine for a variety of articles and information on osteoporosis.

Texas

Since 1995, Texas has required insurers to provide coverage for medically accepted bone mass measurement to detect low bone mass and determine risk of osteoporosis. The Web site is www.tdh.state.tx.us/osteo.

Utah

No current legislation exists.

Vermont

No current legislation exists.

Virginia

In 1995, Virginia initiated an osteoporosis prevention and education program through the Department of Health, in cooperation with the Medical Society of Virginia. The Web site is www.vahealth.org/

nutrition/bones.htm. (Isn't it wonderful to see doctors and government officials working together?)

Washington

In 1990, Washington was one of the first states to deal with osteoporosis when it established the Warren G. Magnuson Institute for Biomedical Research and Health Professions Training to provide research into the causes, treatment, and management of osteoporosis. (Check out www.doh.wa.gov/cfh/osteofin.doc for more info.)

West Virginia

West Virginia created the *Osteoporosis Prevention Education Act* in 1996 and requires the Bureau of Public Health to promote and maintain the program by developing ways to educate the public and health professionals. The state also established the Interagency Council on Osteoporosis to coordinate management of osteoporosis programs. The program's Web site is www.wvdhhr.org/bph/oehp/hp/osteo/default.htm.

Wisconsin

In 1997, Wisconsin provided funding to increase women's awareness of health issues and to reduce chronic and debilitating health problems, such as osteoporosis. Wisconsin's Department of Health and Family Services provides information on osteoporosis at http://dhfs.wisconsin.gov/womenshealth/Osteoporosis.htm.

Wyoming

No current legislation exists.

Glossary

Reading a book about a medical condition can be challenging at times. You often come across terms that seem to reside in a different country, and perhaps even a different planet. We want to ease any confusion you may have by simplifying those terms in this glossary so you aren't left scratching your head and wondering which side is up. Whether you're reading this book or other information about osteoporosis, this section is a short but helpful dictionary that pulls most of the medical terms in *Osteoporosis For Dummies* together.

Note: Any word printed in ***italic and bold type*** has its own definition in its own rightful alphabetical place in this glossary.

Adult rickets: See ***osteomalacia.***

Alendronate (Fosamax): A ***bisphosphonate*** drug used in the treatment of osteoporosis to increase bone mass.

Anorexia nervosa: Excessive fear of being overweight, which results in inadequate food intake.

Baseline measurement: A test or measurement taken before any treatment is begun.

Bisphosphonates: The newest group of medications that improve bone density. Bisphosphonates work to build bone by slowing the removal of bone while allowing more bone to be formed. See ***alendronate, pamidronate, risedronate*** and ***ibandronate sodium.***

Body Mass Index (BMI): A measure of body size that takes into account both height and weight.

Bone: Living, growing tissue made mostly of ***collagen,*** a protein that provides a soft framework, and ***calcium,*** a mineral that adds strength and hardens the framework. The combination of collagen and calcium makes bone strong yet flexible enough to stand up to the abuse you heap on your skeleton every day.

Bone densitometry: A test to detect low bone density. The most common bone density test is called Dual Energy X-ray Absorptiometry ***(DXA test).***

Bone mass: The total amount of bone tissue in the skeleton.

Bone mineral density: The volume of calcium and minerals within the bone tissue; a measurement of bone strength.

Burst fracture: A fracture of the vertebrae that extends through the entire vertebral body. See ***vertebral compression fracture.***

Calcitonin: A hormone secreted by the ***thyroid gland.*** Calcitonin can help slow bone removal, which improves ***bone mineral density.*** It can also help relieve pain associated with fractures. It's available as a medication in two forms: injection or nasal spray.

Calcium: The most abundant mineral in the human body and most important for preventing and treating osteoporosis.

Celiac disease: Also called ***nontropical sprue.*** An inherited intestinal disorder that results in an inability to tolerate *gluten,* a natural protein commonly found in many grains, including wheat, barley, rye, and oats.

Collagen: A protein fiber that comprises a large part of connective tissue (skin and tendons) and bone.

Colles' fracture: A wrist fracture.

Compact bone: See ***cortical bone.***

Cortical bone: Also called ***compact bone.*** The dense outer covering of bone that surrounds ***trabecular bone.*** Found mainly in the appendages.

Corticosteroids: Hormonal steroid substances secreted from the adrenal glands; also a type of steroid drug often used for asthma and rheumatoid arthritis.

Diphosphonates: See ***bisphosphonates.***

Diuretic: A medication or substance that increases urination.

Dowager's hump: An abnormal outward curvature of the upper back with round shoulders and stooped posture caused by bone loss and compression of the vertebrae in the spine in osteoporosis.

DXA test: The gold standard test for measuring bone density, DXA is an abbreviation for Dual Energy X-ray Absorptiometry, a test to evaluate your bone mineral density. DXA uses a very small amount of X-ray to measure bone mass at clinically relevant sites on the body, usually the hip or lumbar spine. The DXA takes only a few minutes to complete and is noninvasive. Doctors use it to diagnose osteoporosis very early before fractures occur.

Elemental calcium: The amount of usable calcium in a calcium supplement.

Endocrine glands: Glands that secrete hormones into the blood.

Esophagitis: Irritation or inflammation of the *esophagus,* the tube that leads from the back of the mouth to the stomach.

Estrogen: A sex hormone that stimulates the development of female secondary sex characteristics. Estrogen levels decline in ***menopause.***

Estrogen replacement therapy (ERT): Drugs given to replace the hormones made by the ovaries before menopause. ERT is a very effective prevention for osteoporosis after ***menopause.***

Etidronate: A bisphosphonate drug used to increase ***bone mass.*** Used in combination with calcium carbonate in Didronal PMO.

Femoral neck: A part of the hipbone that connects the ball of the hip to the long shaft of the thigh bone ***(femur).***

Femur: The thigh bone; the largest bone in the human body.

Fragility fracture: A bone that breaks with minimal or no trauma.

Greater trochanter: Area of bone found at the top part of the ***femur.***

Hemiathroplasty: A partial hip replacement.

Hydroxyapatite: The chief structural component of ***bone,*** composed primarily of calcium phosphate crystals.

Hypercalcemia: High levels of blood calcium.

Hyperparathyroidism: Excessive production of ***parathyroid hormone (PTH)*** disrupting the regulation of ***calcium.*** As a result, calcium is taken from the bones, blood levels of calcium rise, and increased amounts of calcium may be excreted in urine.

Hypogonadism: A decrease in activity of the male/female sex organs resulting in decreased hormone production.

Ibandronate sodium (Boniva): A ***bisphosphonate*** taken once a month to reduce bone loss from osteoporosis.

Idiopathic juvenile osteoporosis: A rare condition where children develop osteoporosis for no known reason.

Inflammatory bowel disease: Inflammation in the small or large intestine.

Kyphoplasty: A treatment for ***vertebral compression fractures.*** A "balloon" is injected into the space between the vertebrae through a catheter. The balloon is then inflated and filled with an orthopedic cement that hardens in place. This helps return the vertebral space to its original height.

Kyphosis: See ***dowager's hump.***

Lordosis: Curvature in the lower spine.

Magnetic Resonance Imaging (MRI): A machine that uses magnetic forces to obtain detailed images of the body.

Malabsorption: The inability to take in adequate amounts of nutrients from the intestinal tract; some forms of malabsorption can cause osteoporosis.

Menopause: The period of natural cessation of menstruation normally occurring between the ages of 45 and 50.

Nontropical sprue: See ***celiac disease.***

Osteoblasts: Cells that form ***bone.***

Osteocalcin: Protein synthesized in bone by active ***osteoblasts.***

Osteoclasts: Cells that break down ***bone.***

Osteocytes: Cells that help maintain ***bone.***

Osteogenesis: The formation of bone in connective tissue or cartilage.

Osteogenesis imperfecta (OI): A genetic disorder characterized by brittle bones that break very easily.

Osteomalacia: A softening of the bones as a result of ***vitamin D*** deficiency. Also known as ***adult rickets.***

Osteopenia: A mild decrease in ***bone mineral density.***

Osteoporosis: A decrease in ***bone mass.*** As the bones become weaker, they become easier to fracture or break. Men as well as women suffer from osteoporosis, a disease that can be prevented and treated.

Osteoprotegerin (OPG): A protein found naturally in the body that reduces the production of ***osteoclasts;*** currently under investigation as a potential osteoporosis treatment.

Pamidronate (Aredia): A ***bisphosphonate*** drug currently under investigation for use with osteoporosis.

Parathyroid hormone (PTH): A hormone under investigation as a treatment for osteoporosis; prevents the level of blood calcium from going too low. Also can stimulate the breakdown of bone. When given intermittently, it can increase ***bone mass.***

Parathyroid hormone or parathomone (PTH): A hormone secreted by the parathyroid gland and associated with calcium utilization in the body.

Peak bone mass: The maximum amount of bone achieved during the years of skeletal growth.

Periosteum: The fibrous membrane covering the outside of ***bone.***

Phosphorus: A mineral active in bone and tissue growth.

Phytoestrogens: An estrogen-like substance found in plants.

Progesterone: A steroid hormone secreted by the ovaries.

Quantitative Computed Tomography (QCT): A test used to measure true ***bone mineral density.***

Raloxifene (Evista): A drug that prevents bone loss; raloxifene is from a new class of drugs called ***Selective Estrogen Receptor Modulators (SERMs).***

Recommended Dietary Allowance (RDA): A U.S. reference for daily nutrient requirements.

Remodeling: The process of replacing old bone with new bone through the action of ***osteoclasts*** and ***osteoblasts.***

Resistance-type exercises: Exercises where muscle is acting against resistance, such as weight lifting.

Resorption: The breakdown and assimilation of bone through the action of ***osteoclasts.***

Rickets: A childhood disease resulting in soft, weak bones, caused by lack of vitamin D, calcium, or phosphate.

Risedronate (Actonel): A ***bisphosphonate*** for the prevention and treatment of osteoporosis.

Selective Estrogen Receptor Modulators (SERMs): Drugs used to prevent osteoporosis in postmenopausal women. SERMs act like ***estrogen*** in some tissues, and block the effects of estrogen in others, which is why they're called "selective."

Spongy bone: See ***trabecular bone.***

Standard Deviation (SD): A consistent unit of measure above or below the average of a comparison group.

Strontium ranelate (Protelos): Strontium ranelate stimulates the formation of new bone tissue and decreases bone loss; available in Europe for treatment of osteoporosis.

T-Score: Osteoporosis experts consider normal bone density to be that of a normal, young adult. In the ***DXA test,*** this measurement is called a normal "T-score." A T-score of –1.0 or higher is in the normal range. A score between –1.0 and –2.0 means that your bone density is borderline for osteoporosis (osteopenia). A T-score of –2.0 or lower qualifies as osteoporosis.

Teriparatide (rhPTH) (Forteo): A *recombinant* (manmade) form of the active part of ***parathyroid hormone.*** Used to treat osteoporosis by increasing bone mass and strength.

Testosterone: The major male sex hormone.

Thyroid gland: Part of the ***endocrine system,*** found at the front of the neck. Secretes hormones that are important for normal body growth and metabolism.

Tibolone (Livial): A synthetic steroid that mimics the activity of estrogen and progesterone (female sex hormones) in the body.

Trabecular bone: Also called ***spongy bone,*** trabecular bone is a honeycomblike structure of bony tissue.

Ultrasound: High frequency sound waves used to image internal structures of the body.

Vertebrae: The bony segments of the spinal column.

Vertebral compression fracture: An injury to the spine in which one or more vertebrae collapse. If the collapse is only in the front part of the spine, it's called a compression fracture or ***wedge fracture.*** If the vertebral body is crushed in all directions, it's called a ***burst fracture.***

Vertebroplasty: A procedure to treat compression fractures. Orthopedic cement is injected into the space between the vertebrae; as it hardens the vertebral space is restored to its original height.

Vitamin D: Essential vitamin that allows the bones to absorb ***calcium.*** Vitamin D allows calcium to leave the intestine and enter the bloodstream.

Wedge fracture: A ***vertebral compression fracture*** occurring at the front or the back of the vertebrae only; the collapse at one end or the other of the vertebrae looks like a wedge.

Weight-bearing exercise: Exercise in which a person supports his or her own body weight, such as walking.

Z-score: Measures standard deviations for a specific group. A Z-score from a ***DXA test*** compares a person to controls matched for age, weight, gender, and race.

Zoledronic acid (Zometa): Used to treat ***hypercalcemia.***

Index

• A •

AAMA (American Academy of Medical Acupuncture), 189
acetaminophen (Tylenol), 17, 182
acidity, 83
acidosis, 64
acrylic cement, 208, 220
Activators of Non-Genomic Estrogen-Like Signaling (ANGELS), 219
Actonel. *See* risedronate
acupressure, 190
acupuncture, 189
addiction, pain medication, 186–187
adult rickets, 263. *See also* osteomalacia
Advil. *See* ibuprofen
AEDs (anti-epileptic drugs), 46
age
  calcium requirement, 72, 73
  effect on building bone, 233
  recommended vitamin D intake and, 163
  as risk factor for osteoporosis, 35
Alabama, osteoporosis program, 251
Alaska, osteoporosis program, 251
alcohol consumption
  effects of, 15, 41–42, 56, 83–84, 233
  helping teens to avoid, 250
Aleeve (naproxen), 17, 183
alendronate (Fosamax)
  definition, 263
  dose, 149–150
  Food and Drug Administration approval, 58
  risedronate compared, 246
  use, 148
  vitamin D levels and, 164
aluminum, 174
amenorrhea, 85
American Academy of Medical Acupuncture (AAMA), 189
American College of Rheumatology (Web site), 185, 214, 242
American Massage Therapy Association (AMTA), 190
American Medical Association (AMA), 34, 35
American Psychiatric Society, 60
American Society for Bone and Mineral Research (ASBMR), 214
amitriptylene (antidepressant), 185
androgen-deprivation therapy, for prostate cancer, 58–59
androgens, 58, 160
andropause, 56
anesthesia, 201
ANGELS (Activators of Non-Genomic Estrogen-Like Signaling), 219
anorexia nervosa
  definition, 60, 263
  as risk factor for osteoporosis, 37
  treatment, 61
  watching for, 249
antacids, 174
antibiotics, 202, 203
antidepressants (amitriptylene), 185
anti-epileptic drugs (AEDs), 46
anti-HIV drugs, 47
antiresorptive drugs, 147
aquatic physical therapy, 188
Aredia. *See* pamidronate
Arizona, osteoporosis program, 252
Arkansas, osteoporosis program, 252
arthritis
  osteoarthritis, 16–17, 198, 244–245
  rheumatoid, 49
  wrist fracture and, 210
arthroplasty, 198
artificial hip joints. *See* hip replacement
ASBMR (American Society for Bone and Mineral Research), 214
aspirin, 17, 183, 184, 203

Association of Rheumatology Health Professionals, 241
astronauts, osteoporosis and, 51
avascular necrosis, 198

• B •

back pain
  idiopathic juvenile osteoporosis (IJO), 65
  osteoporosis and, 245
  from vertebral compression fractures, 115, 116, 179
back.com (Web site), 208
baseline measurement, 263
beans, as calcium source, 75
beta-carotene, 166–167
Bextra, 184
biceps curls with dumbbells (exercise), 95–96
binge eating, 61
biochemical markers of bone turnover, 139
biofeedback, 191
bisphosphonates
  contraindications, 149
  correct use of, 149–150
  description, 147, 263
  intravenous, 158–159, 219
  mode of action, 148
  new ways of giving, 219
  to offset antihormone drugs, 59
  for osteogenesis imperfecta, 65
  research on, 219
  side effects, 149, 219
  when to use, 148–149
blood cells, production of, 20
blood clots, 154, 202, 203
blood pressure, high, 108
blood tests, of bone turnover, 139
body mass index (BMI)
  body weight relationship, 37–39
  definition, 264
bone
  collagen in, 24
  definition, 263
  functions, 20–21
  hormone effects on, 26–28
  minerals and bone growth, 28–29
  modeling, 24
  number in human body, 21
  remodeling, 10, 24–26, 235, 268
  sesmoid, 21
  structure, 22–24
  types, 22
  wormian, 21
Bone and Joint Decade (Web site), 221
bone biopsy
  location for, 18
  osteomalacia diagnosis, 17, 18
  in secondary hyperparathyroidism, 49
bone density
  measurements by age, sex, and race, 30
  reduction in osteopenia, 18
bone density testing (bone densitometry)
  accuracy of, 134
  baseline, 67
  blood and urine tests, 139
  description, 12, 134, 245, 263
  DXA (Dual Energy X-Ray Absorptiometry), 136–137
  frequency of, 143
  interpreting results of, 139–143
  markers of bone turnover, 139
  Medicare coverage, 128–129, 136
  PDXA (Peripheral Dual Energy X-Ray Absorptiometry), 138
  pQCT (Peripheral Quantitative Computed Tomography), 138
  RA (Radiographic Absorptiometry), 138
  SXA (Single Energy X-Ray Absorptiometry), 137
  T-score, 140–141
  ultrasound, 139
  when to have, 134–135
  X-rays compared, 134
  Z-score, 141–142
bone marrow, 20
bone mass
  definition, 264
  density, 41
  peak, 13–15, 29–30, 267

bone mineral density
baseline scan, 55
definition, 264
bone resorption
calcitonin effect on, 41
definition, 268
osteoclasts and, 26
remodeling and, 24, 26
vitamin A effect on, 46
bone specific alkaline phosphatase (BSAP), 139
Boning Up On Osteoporosis (National Osteoporosis Foundation), 237
Boniva. *See* ibandronate
braces
fitting by occupational therapist, 210
for pain management, 190
spinal fractures and, 208, 210
Thoracic-Lumbar-Sacral Orthosis (TLSO), 208
breast cancer, 150, 157
breast milk, 64
Brizer, David, MD (*Quitting Smoking For Dummies*), 41, 233
Building Strength Together (BST) support group, 237–238, 239
bulimia nervosa
description, 61–62
as risk factor for osteoporosis, 37
burst fracture, 207, 264

• C •

C teleopeptide (CTX), 139
caffeine
in Excedrin, 84
interaction with calcium, 84–85, 170
urine output and, 43
calcitonin
alcohol effect on, 41
definition, 264
forms of medication, 155
functions of, 27–28
for pain management, 155, 185, 208
side effects, 155
calcium
daily requirement, 50, 56, 72, 167, 244
definition, 264
elemental, 168–169, 265
in hydroxyapatite, 24, 28
hypercalciuria, 37, 49
on nutritional labels, 79
storage in bone, 21, 28, 234
calcium carbonate, 168–172, 174
calcium citrate, 168–169, 170, 172, 243
calcium gluconate, 168–169
calcium lactate, 168–169
calcium sources
beans, 75
chocolate cake, 230
dairy, 74–75
fruits, 75
latte, 229
milk, 43, 74, 232–233, 244
mineral water, 227–228
molasses, 76, 230
nuts, 75, 228–229
orange juice, 75, 229
pizza, 229
powdered milk, 230
seeds, 75, 228–229
tables of, 74–76
tacos, 229
vegetables, 78, 228
calcium supplements
antacid tablets, 174
best, 243
caveats on taking, 169–170
combinations with other vitamins and minerals, 173
description, 167–168
dissolvability, 171–172
elemental calcium, 168–169, 265
interactions with foods and medications, 170–171
lead content, 172
medical conditions affected by, 175
California, osteoporosis program, 252
canaliculi, 26
cancer
breast, 150, 157
endometrial, 159
liver, 157
prostate cancer, 55, 56, 58–59, 158
skin, 163
uterine, 150, 151

capitation, 131
carbonated drinks, avoiding, 249
carpal tunnel syndrome, 210
celecoxib (Celebrex), 183, 184
celiac disease
  bone loss and, 48
  in children, 64
  definition, 264
cement, 199, 208, 209, 220
Centers for Disease Control (CDC), 113
chatroom, 239–240
cheese, 75, 77
children
  anorexia nervosa, 60–61, 249
  breastfeeding, 64
  bulimia, 61–62
  calcium intake, 72, 73
  calcium needs, 15
  carbonated drinks, avoiding, 249
  cigarettes and alcohol, avoiding, 250
  corticosteroids, 66–67
  dieting and bone loss, 60–62
  exercise, 15, 88, 247
  family history, knowing, 250
  female athlete triad, 62–63
  idiopathic juvenile osteoporosis, 54, 63, 65
  lactose intolerance, 248–249
  milk consumption, 248
  osteogenesis imperfecta, 24, 50, 64–66, 266
  rickets, 63–64
  setting an example for, 250
  shopping wisely for, 248
chiropractors, acupuncture by, 189
chocolate cake, as calcium source, 230
collagen
  definition, 264
  osteogenesis imperfecta and, 24, 50, 65
  production by osteoblasts, 25
  as structural component of bone, 24
collagenase, 25
Colles' fracture, 37, 109–110, 210, 264
Colorado, osteoporosis program, 252
Commission for Massage Training Accreditation (COMTA), 190
compact bone, 264. *See also* cortical bone
compression fracture, 114–117. *See also* vertebral compression fractures
compression stockings, 203
computed tomography (CT) scan
  compression fracture diagnosis, 207
  helical (volumetric) CT scanning, 217
  hip fracture diagnosis, 198
  Peripheral Quantitative Computed Tomography (pQCT), 138
Connecticut, osteoporosis program, 253
connective tissue disease, 49
co-pay, insurance, 131
coral calcium, 171
cortical bone
  definition, 22, 264
  healing time, 212
  location, 22–23
  loss of, 23
  remodeling and, 24
corticosteroids
  bone densitometry recommendations and, 143
  in children, 66–67
  definition, 264
  effect on bone, 44–45
  inhaled, 66–67
  in men, 56–57
  precautions, 44–45
  preventive therapy while using, 156
  side effects, 44
  treating corticosteroid-induced osteoporosis, 67
cortisol, 61
Coumadin (warfarin), 174, 184, 203
COX (cyclooxygenase) enzymes, 183, 184
creatinine, 67
Crohn's disease, 47

Cross-Training For Dummies (Tony Ryan and Martica Heaner), 104
crutches, 199–200, 205
CT scan. *See* computed tomography (CT) scan
CTX (C teleopeptide), 139
Cushing's syndrome, 45, 57
cyclooxygenase (COX) enzymes, 183, 184
cytokines, 49

• D •

dairy products
- calcium content, 74–75
- lactose content, 77

deep vein thrombosis (DVT), 203
degenerative joint disease, 17
Delaware, osteoporosis program, 253
deltoid muscles, 98
densitometry. *See* bone density testing (bone densitometry)
depression, 125
designer estrogens, 154–155
DHEA (steroid hormone), 58
diagnosis
- future technologies for, 217
- importance of early, 13–14

diet
- acid nutrients, 83
- alcohol, 83–84
- caffeine, 84–85
- calcium, 72–79
- eating healthy, 250
- food labels, 79, 248
- fracture healing and, 205
- honesty with doctor concerning, 126
- lactose intolerance, 76–77
- nutritional labels, 79
- phosphorus, 81
- potassium, 82
- protein, 82–83
- as risk factor for osteoporosis, 42–43
- sodium, 82
- vegetables, 78
- vitamin D, 80–81

dieting and bone loss
- anorexia nervosa, 60–61
- bulimia, 61–62
- female athlete triad, 62–63

digital rectal exam, 59
dilantin, 170
diphosphonates, 264. *See also* bisphosphonates
disc degeneration, 116
District of Columbia, osteoporosis program, 253
diuretics
- definition, 264
- for hypercalciuria treatment, 37

doctors
- choosing a specialist, 120–121
- educating, 215–216
- encouraging patients to change habits, 214
- family, 120
- find the right doctor, 124
- first appointment, preparing for, 123–124
- follow-up appointments with, 127–128
- honesty with, 126–127
- metabolic bone specialists, 121–122
- questions to ask, 122–123
- as resource, 241
- treatment plan setup, 124–125

dowager's hump
- appearance of, 114, 115
- cause, 114, 115, 220
- definition, 264
- kyphoplasty and, 190, 209, 220–221

drugs
- acetaminophen (Tylenol), 17, 182
- alendronate (Fosamax), 58, 148–150, 164, 246, 263
- amitriptylene (antidepressant), 185
- antibiotics, 202, 203
- anti-epileptic drugs (AEDs), 46
- anti-HIV drugs, 47
- aspirin, 17, 183, 184, 203
- Bextra, 184

drugs *(continued)*
bisphosphonates, 69, 147–150, 158–159, 219, 263
celecoxib (Celebrex), 183, 184
Estren (synthetic estrogen), 219
etidronate, 265
Excedrin, 84
gabapentin (Neurontin), 185, 191
heparin, 46, 203
ibandronate (Boniva), 148, 150, 266
ibuprofen (Motrin and Advil), 17, 183, 184
leuprolide acetate (Lupron), 46, 59
naproxen (Aleeve), 17, 183
NSAID (nonsteroidal anti-inflammatory drug), 182–184
pamidronate (Aredia), 65, 158, 219, 267
raloxifene (Evista), 154–155, 267
risedronate (Actonel), 148–149, 164, 246, 268
strontium ranelate (Protelos), 159–160, 268
teriparatide (rhPTH) (Forteo), 268
teripeptide, 156
tetracycline, 171
tibolone (Livial), 160, 269
Vioxx, 183, 184
warfarin (Coumadin), 174, 184, 203
zoledronic acid (Zometa), 158–159, 219, 269
Dual Energy X-Ray Absorptiometry (DXA)
anorexia nervosa and, 61
baseline, 124
description, 12, 136–137, 265
helical (volumetric CT scanning) compared, 217
idiopathic juvenile osteoporosis (IJO), 65
limitations of, 217
Medicare coverage of, 128–129
Peripheral Dual Energy X-Ray Absorptiometry (PDXA), 138
results, interpretation of, 139–143
DVT (deep vein thrombosis), 203

• E •

eating. *See* diet
Ehler-Danlos syndrome, 49
elemental calcium, 168, 265
Eli Lilly (Web site), 242
endocrine glands
definition, 265
parathyroid gland, overactive, 50
thyroid gland, 27, 50, 268
endocrinologist, 121
endometrial cancer
study for, 159
uterine cancer and, 150, 151
endorphins, 188
ERT. *See* estrogen replacement therapy
esophagitis
bisphosphonates and, 149, 150, 158, 219
definition, 265
reflux, 158
Estren (synthetic estrogen), 219
estrogen
definition, 265
drugs that lower, 46
Estren, 219
fat cell production of, 40
function of, 28
loss in menopause, 10, 31
phytoestrogen, 220, 267
smoking effect on, 40
ultra low-dose estrogen, 159
estrogen replacement therapy (ERT)
correct use of, 151–153
definition, 265
designer estrogens, 154–155
FDA approval, 150
patches, 153
pills, combination, 152–153
pills, estrogen-only, 152
for postmenopausal symptoms, 150
side effects, 150–151, 153–154
smoking effect on, 41
etidronate, 265
Evista (raloxifene), 154–155, 267
Excedrin, 84

Exercise: A Video from the National Institute on Aging, 104
exercise and exercising
after hip replacement, 203
after vertebral fracture, 209
aquatic, 188
best for preventing osteoporosis, 244
building bone with, 89–90
children, 15, 88, 247
effect on menstrual periods, 37
finding time for, 92
honesty with doctor concerning, 126
injury, avoiding, 92–93
by men, 56
for pain management, 188
plan, 125
questions to ask concerning, 9
resistance training, 89, 90, 94, 268
routine, 93–94
schedule, setting, 91–92
starting when young, 88
weight-bearing, 89–90, 244, 269
exercises
biceps curls with dumbbells, 95–96
hip extensors, 100–101
hip flexors, 101–102
knee extensors, 99–100
leg lifts, 103–104
overhead press, 98–99
triceps kickback, 96–97
extracapsular fractures, 198, 199

• F •

falls
hip fractures and, 112–113
hip protectors, 196
postural instability, 113
preventing, 194–196
reducing with vitamin D, 165
family history
future research on understanding role of, 218
knowing, 15, 249
as risk factor for osteoporosis, 35–37, 218
fat cells, estrogen production by, 40
female athlete triad, 15, 62–63
femoral neck, 111, 265
femur
definition, 265
fracture of, 111–113
Fitness Over Forty For Dummies (Betsy Nagelsen McCormack and Mike Yorkey), 240
flat bones, 22
Florida, osteoporosis program, 253
Food and Drug Administration (FDA)
alendronate and, 58
ibandronate and, 150
limits on lead in calcium supplements, 172
pamidronate and, 219
raloxifene and, 154
food labels, 79, 248
Forteo (teriparatide) (rhPTH), 268
Fosamax. *See* alendronate
fractures. *See also specific fractures*
bracing, 190
calcium intake for prevention of, 232
checking for osteoporosis after, 194
cost to society, 234
falls and, 194–196
fragility, 12, 17, 108–110, 215–216, 265
greenstick, 29
healing time, 211
hip, 12, 54–55, 111–113, 197–206
lifetime risk by gender, table of, 108
mortality rate and, 112, 232
multiple, 109
pain and, 178–180, 231
pelvic, 211
reducing chance of future, 212
ribs, 211
statistics, 11–12, 35
stress, 113
vertebral compression, 11–12, 114–117, 206–210, 220–221, 269
wedge, 114, 115, 207, 269
wrist (Colles'), 12, 109–110, 197, 210
fragility fracture
description, 12, 108–109, 265
doctor education on, 215–216

fragility fracture *(continued)*
osteogenesis imperfecta and, 109
osteomalacia and, 17, 109, 216
wrist fracture as, 110
fruits, as calcium source, 75
Fuentes, Manny (*T'ai Chi For Dummies*), 210

• G •

gabapentin (Neurontin), 185, 191
gastrointestinal diseases, 47–48
gender
anorexia and, 61
fracture risk, 108
hip fractures and, 54–55
as osteoporosis risk factor, 34
genetics. *See* family history
Georgia, osteoporosis program, 254
geriatrician, 121
gluten, 48
gonadomimetic, 160
Got Milk? campaign, 74, 242
Grave's disease, 45
greater trochanter, 265
greenstick fracture, 29
guided imagery, 191
gyms, 93
gynecologist, 121

• H •

Harvard Medical School, 165, 239
Hashimoto's disease, 45
Hawaii, osteoporosis program, 254
health maintenance organization (HMO), 129, 130
Heaner, Martica (*Cross-Training For Dummies*), 104
heat packs, 187
height loss
causes of, 116
health effects of, 233–234
with scoliosis, 116, 246
vertebral compression fractures and, 11, 36, 114, 115
helical CT scanning, 217
hemiathroplasty
definition, 265
partial hip replacement, 198
heparin, 46, 203
heredity. *See* family history
heterogeneous disease, 218
hip dislocation, 202
hip extensors (exercise), 100–101
hip flexors (exercise), 100–101
hip fracture
consequences of, 111–112
description, 111
diagnosis, 197–198
falling and, 112–113
hospital stay, 201–202
location of fracture, 198
in men and women, 54–55
mortality rate, effect on, 112, 232
physical activity after hip surgery, 203–205
planning for surgery and aftercare, 199–200
postoperative care, 202–203
revision surgery, 206
statistics, 11, 12, 35, 111, 197
vitamin D deficiency and, 165
hip protectors, 196
hip replacement
cemented prosthesis, 198
complications, 202–203
how long they last, 206
incision size, 201
length of surgery, 201
partial (hemiathroplasty), 198
physical activity after, 203
revision surgery, 206
total (arthoplasty), 198
hiprotector.com (Web site), 196
HMO (health maintenance organization), 129, 130
hormone replacement therapy (HRT), 150. *See also* estrogen replacement therapy (ERT)
hormones affecting bone. *See also specific hormones*
calcitonin, 27–28
estrogen, 28

parathyroid hormone (PTH), 27
testosterone, 28
vitamin D, 27
hospitalization, for hip surgery, 201–202
HRT (hormone replacement therapy), 150. *See also* estrogen replacement therapy (ERT)
humerus, 109
hydroxyapatite
components of, 24, 28
definition, 265
osteoclast action on, 25
hypercalcemia, 265
hypercalciuria, 37, 49
hypermobility of joints, 49
hyperparathyroidism
calcium supplements and, 175
definition, 265
as risk factor for osteoporosis, 57
secondary, 49
hypertension, 108
hyperthyroid, 45
hypnosis, 191
hypogonadism
definition, 266
in men, 56, 57
hypothyroid, 45
hysterectomy, 151, 152

• I •

ibandronate (Boniva)
definition, 266
difficulty in locating, 148
dosage, 150
Food and Drug Administration (FDA) approval, 150
ibuprofen (Motrin and Advil), 17, 183, 184
ice packs, 187–188
Idaho, osteoporosis program, 254
idiopathic juvenile osteoporosis (IJO)
description, 54, 63, 266
diagnosis and treatment, 65
Iknoian, Therese (*T'ai Chi For Dummies*), 210
iliac crest, bone biopsy and, 18
Illinois, osteoporosis program, 254
Indiana, osteoporosis program, 254
infection, post-surgery, 202, 203
inflammatory bowel disease, 47, 266
injury, avoiding while exercising, 92–93
insurance
appeals, 130–131
capitation, 131
communicating with provider, 128
co-pay, 131
drug coverage, 131
health maintenance organization (HMO), 129, 130
Medicare, 128–129
out of network referral, 131
Point of Service (POS), 130
Preferred Provider Organization (PPO), 130
state-mandated coverage, 129
International Congress on Osteoporosis, 222
International Dairy Foods, 242
International Osteoporosis Foundation (IOF)
projects, 221–222
recommendations on vertebral body fractures, 115
Web site, 221–222
International Society of Bone Densitometry, 143
International Society of Clinical Densitometry, 121
intertrochanteric fractures, 198
intracapsular fractures, 198
Iowa, osteoporosis program, 255
iron, interaction with calcium, 170
irregular bones, 22

• J •

juice
calcium-fortified, 249
orange, 75, 229
juvenile epiphysitis (Scheuermann's disease), 116
juvenile rheumatoid arthritis, 49

• K •

Kaiser Family Foundation, 130
Kansas, osteoporosis program, 255
Kentucky, osteoporosis program, 255
kidney disease
  chronic, effects of, 49
  renal osteodystrophy, 49
  rickets and, 64
kidney stones, 49, 175
knee extensors (exercise), 99–100
kyphoplasty
  complications, 209, 221
  definition, 266
  dowager's hump and, 190, 209, 220–221
  procedure, 190, 208, 220–221
  vertebroplasty compared, 209, 221
kyphosis, 114, 207, 266. *See also* dowager's hump

• L •

Lactaid, 77
lactase, 76
lactose intolerance
  children, 248–249
  living with, 76–77
  race and, 76
latte, as calcium source, 229
laxative, interaction with calcium, 170
lead, in calcium supplements, 172–173
leg lifts (exercise), 103–104
legislation, state osteoporosis, 251–261
leuprolide acetate (Lupron), 46, 59
lidocaine, 185
lifestyle factors, in osteoporosis, 40–43
liver disease
  cancer, 157
  cirrhosis, 49
  rickets and, 64
  testosterone replacement therapy and, 58
Livial (tibolone), 160, 269
long bones, 22
lordosis, 266
Louisiana, osteoporosis program, 255
low-density lipoprotein receptor protein 5, 218
Lupron (leuprolide acetate), 46, 59

• M •

magnesium
  alcohol effect on, 42
  effect on calcium absorption, 171
  storage in bone, 234
Maine, osteoporosis program, 255
malabsorption, definition, 266
markers, of bone turnover, 139
Maryland, osteoporosis program, 255
Massachusetts, osteoporosis program, 256
massage therapy, 190
Mayo Clinic (Web site), 239
McCormack, Betsy Nagelsen (*Fitness Over Forty For Dummies*), 240
Medicare, 128–129, 131, 136
medications. *See also specific drugs*
  bisphosphonates, 147–150, 158–159, 219
  bone loss from, 43–47
  calcitonin, 155
  combination drug therapies, 159
  discussing with doctor, 125
  estrogen replacement, 150–155, 159, 219
  future, 218–220
  generic and brand names, table of, 146–147
  honesty with doctor concerning, 127
  insurance coverage, 131
  new directions in, 158–160
  noncompliance with, 218
  OTC pain medicines, 181–184
  preventive therapy, 156
  research, 218–220
  strontium, 159–160
  teripeptides, 156

testosterone replacement, 157–158
tibolone (Livial), 160
medlineplus.com (Web site), 242
medscape.com (Web site), 242
men, osteoporosis in
andropause, 56
hip fractures, 54–55, 56
Mr. OS study, 55–56
prevention, 59
prostate cancer and, 58–59
risk factors, 57
statistics on, 53–54
treatment, 57–58, 59
menopause
alcohol effect on, 42
definition, 266
estrogen decrease and, 10, 31
estrogen replacement therapy, 150
smoking effect on, 41
menstrual periods
age at start and stopping of, 40
amenorrhea, 85
anorexia nervosa and, 60, 61
effect of exercise and diet on, 37
Merck (Web site), 242
metabolic bone disease, 109
metabolic bone specialists, 121–122
methyl methacrylate, 199
Michigan, osteoporosis program, 223, 256
milk
breast, 64
as calcium source, 43, 74, 232–233, 244
consumption by children, 248
Got Milk? campaign, 74
as vitamin D source, 80
Milk Matters program, 222
mineral water, as calcium source, 227–228
Minnesota, osteoporosis program, 256
Mississippi, osteoporosis program, 256
Missouri, osteoporosis program, 256
modeling, 24
molasses, as calcium source, 76, 230
Montana, osteoporosis program, 257
Motrin. *See* ibuprofen
Mr. OS study, 55–56
MRI (magnetic resonance imaging)
compression fracture diagnosis, 207
definition, 266
hip fracture diagnosis, 198
multiple myeloma, 49–50
multivitamins, 173
music therapy, 191

• N •

N teleopeptide (NTX), 139
naproxen (Aleeve), 17, 183
National Certification Commission for Acupuncture and Oriental Medicine (NCCAOM), 189
National Committee for Quality Assurance, 222
National Health and Nutrition Examination Survey (NHANES), 30
National Institute on Aging
Exercise: A Video from the National Institute on Aging, 104, 240
Web site, 104, 240
National Institute on Aging and National Cancer Institute, 55
National Institute on Aging Information Center (NIAIC), 238
National Institutes of Health (NIH)
acupuncture and, 189
Milk Matters program, 222
Web site, 222
women's Health Initiative Memory study, 151
National Jewish Medical and Research Center, 66
National Osteoporosis Foundation (NOF)
Boning Up On Osteoporosis, 237
Building Strength Together (BST) support group, 237–238, 239

National Osteoporosis Foundation *(continued)*
on cost of osteoporotic fractures, 234
Osteoporosis Report, 237
osteoporosis statistics, 34
recommendations on when to have a bone density test, 135
Web site, 214, 237–238
naturopaths, acupuncture by, 189
NCCAOM (National Certification Commission for Acupuncture and Oriental Medicine), 189
Nebraska, osteoporosis program, 257
Neporent, Liz (*Weight Training For Dummies*), 104, 240
Neurontin (gabapentin), 185
Nevada, osteoporosis program, 257
New Hampshire, osteoporosis program, 257
New Jersey, osteoporosis program, 223, 257
New Mexico, osteoporosis program, 258
New York, osteoporosis program, 258
NHANES (National Health and Nutrition Examination Survey), 30
NIAIC (National Institute on Aging Information Center), 238
NIH. *See* National Institutes of Health
NIH National Institute of Arthritis and Musculoskeletal and Skin Diseases (NIAMS), 55
NIH Osteoporosis and Related Bone Diseases-National Resource Center (Web site), 238
NOF. *See* National Osteoporosis Foundation
nontropical sprue, 266. *See also* celiac disease
North Carolina, osteoporosis program, 223, 258
North Dakota, osteoporosis program, 258
novocaine, 185
NSAID (nonsteroidal anti-inflammatory drug), 182–184
NTX (N teleopeptide), 139
nursing homes
falls by patients in, 194
hip fractures and, 112, 232
nutritional labels, 79
nuts, as calcium source, 75, 228–229

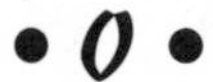

obesity, 85–86
oblique muscles, 98
occupational therapists, 204, 205
occupational therapy, 210
Ohio, osteoporosis program, 258
OI. *See* osteogenesis imperfecta
Oklahoma, osteoporosis program, 258–259
online resources, 241–242
OPG. *See* osteoprotegerin
orange juice, as calcium source, 75, 229
Oregon, osteoporosis program, 259
orthopedic surgeon, 121
osteoarthritis
description, 16–17
distinguishing pain from hip fractures, 198
osteoporosis compared, 244–245
osteoblasts
alcohol effect on, 42
cytokine effects on, 50
definition, 266
functions, 25–26, 28
osteoprotegerin (OPG) production by, 26, 220
osteocalcin
as bone formation marker, 139
corticosteroids and, 67
definition, 266
osteoclasts
activation by osteoprotegerin (OPG), 26, 220
alcohol effect on, 42
bisphosphonates and, 147, 148
collagenase production by, 25

cytokine effects on, 49
definition, 266
function, 25–26, 28
osteocalcin and, 67
research on, 220
osteocytes
definition, 266
osteoblasts and, 25–26
osteogenesis, definition, 266
osteogenesis imperfecta (OI)
casts and, 66
cause, 24, 50, 65
definition, 266
features of, 65
hereditary nature of, 64
treatment, 65
osteomalacia
after stomach surgery, 48
compression fractures and, 116
description, 24, 267
diagnosis, 15, 17, 18, 48
fragility fractures and, 17, 109, 216
osteoporosis compared, 17–18
rickets, 63
vitamin D deficiency and, 164
osteonecrosis, 198
osteo.org (Web site), 238
osteopenia
bone density and, 18
definition, 18, 267
diagnosis, 18
risk factors, 57
osteoporosis
aging, relationship to, 13
definition, 9–10, 267
statistics on, 11–12
Osteoporosis Report (National Osteoporosis Foundation), 237
osteoprotegerin (OPG)
definition, 267
osteoclast activation by, 26, 220
phytoestrogen effect on, 220
production by osteoblasts, 26, 220
OTC pain medicines, 181–184
overhead press (exercise), 98–99
oxalic acid, 78, 171

• P •

Paget's disease, 158, 219
pain
idiopathic juvenile osteoporosis (IJO), 65
osteoporosis and, 17, 245
rickets, 63
from vertebral compression fractures, 115, 116, 179
pain management
acupressure, 190
acupuncture, 190
acute pain, 180–185
addiction, 186–187
back pain, 179
braces, 190
chronic pain, 185–187
dizziness/wooziness from, 185–186
exercise, 188
heat and ice packs, 187–188
kyphoplasty for, 208–209
massage therapy, 190
multiple medications, 186
narcotics, 180–181
nonmedication methods, 187–191
NSAIDs, 181–184
OTC medicines, 181–184
physical therapy, 188
psychological, 190–191
recognizing pain, 178, 179
specialists in, 191
TENS units, 189
pamidronate (Aredia)
definition, 267
dose and frequency of administration, 158, 219
Food and Drug Administration and, 219
intravenous delivery, 65, 158, 219
in patients with esophagitis, 158, 219
side effects, 158
parathyroid gland, overactive, 50
parathyroid hormone (PTH)
alcohol effect on, 42
definition, 267

parathyroid hormone *(continued)*
  disadvantages, 156
  functions of, 27
  uses, 156
parenting tips
  anorexia, watching for, 249
  carbonated drinks, avoiding, 249
  cigarettes and alcohol, avoiding, 250
  exercise, 247
  family history, knowing, 250
  lactose intolerance, 248–249
  milk consumption, 248
  setting an example, 250
  shopping wisely, 248
PDXA (Peripheral Dual Energy X-Ray Absorptiometry), 138
peak bone mass
  age and, 13, 15, 29–30
  definition, 267
  improving, 14–15
pelvic fractures, 211
Pennsylvania, osteoporosis program, 259
percutaneous vertebroplasty, 190, 208
periosteum, definition, 267
Peripheral Dual Energy X-Ray Absorptiometry (PDXA), 138
Peripheral Quantitative Computed Tomography (pQCT), 138
phosphoric acid, 43, 84, 249
phosphorus
  daily intake, 81
  definition, 267
  effect on calcium absorption, 171
  excess in diet, 29
  in hydroxyapatite, 28
  kidney disease and, 49
  storage in bone, 21, 29, 234
photodensitometry, 138
physiatrists, 121
physical therapist
  Association of Rheumatology Health Professionals, 241
  as resource, 241
  role of, 204–205
physical therapy
  after hip surgery, 203–205
  after wrist fracture, 210
  aquatic, 188
  for pain management, 188
  vertebral fractures and, 209
phytoestrogens
  definition, 267
  osteoprotegerin and, 220
pizza, as calcium source, 229
plasma cells, 49
pneumonia, 202, 203
polycythemia, 58, 158
POS (Point of Service), 130
postural instability, 113
potassium, 82
powdered milk, as calcium source, 230
PPO (Preferred Provider Organization), 130
pQCT (Peripheral Quantitative Computed Tomography), 138
prednisone, 44, 66, 156
prevention, osteoporosis
  improving, 213–217
  research, 216–217
  therapy, 156
Procter & Gamble (Web site), 242
progesterone
  definition, 267
  estrogen replacement therapy and, 150–151, 152
prognosis, 125
prostate cancer, 55, 56, 58–59, 158
prostate specific antigen (PSA), 59
prosthesis, hip, 198–199, 206
protein, dietary, 43, 82–83
Protelos. *See* strontium ranelate
PTH. *See* parathyroid hormone

• Q •

quantitative computed tomography (QCT), 267
questions
  to ask doctors, 122–123
  concerning exercise and exercising, 9
  patients ask about osteoporosis, 243–246
Quitting Smoking For Dummies (David Brizer, MD), 41, 233

• R •

race
  lactose intolerance, 76
  osteoporosis and, 36, 54
  vitamin D deficiency and, 163
Radiographic Absorptiometry (RA), 138
radius, 109
raloxifene (Evista), 154–155, 267
recommended dietary allowance (RDA), 73, 267
relaxation training, 191
remodeling
  continual nature of, 10, 235
  definition, 268
  process description, 24–26
renal osteodystrophy, 49
research
  on medications, 218–220
  ongoing, 223
  in osteoporosis prevention, 216–217
resistance training, 89–90, 94, 268
resorption markers, 139
resorption of bone
  calcitonin effect on, 41
  definition, 268
  osteoclasts and, 26
  remodeling and, 24, 26
  vitamin A effect on, 46
resources. *See also* Web sites
  books, 240
  chatroom, 240
  doctor, 241
  Harvard Medical School, 239
  Mayo Clinic, 239
  National Institutes of Health (NIH), 238
  National Osteoporosis Foundation (NOF), 238–239
  online, 241–242
  physical therapist, 241
  support groups, 239, 240
  videos, 240
retinol, 166
revision surgery, 206
rheumatoid arthritis, 49
rheumatologist, 17, 120–121, 158, 242
rheumatology, 213
rheumatology.org (Web site), 17, 242
Rhode Island, osteoporosis program, 259
rhPTH (teriparatide), 268
ribs
  collapse in idiopathic juvenile osteoporosis, 65
  fractures, 211
rickets. *See also* osteomalacia
  causes and effects, 63–64
  definition, 268
risedronate (Actonel)
  alendronate compared, 246
  definition, 268
  dose, 149
  use, 148
  vitamin D levels, 164
risk factors
  age, 35
  alcohol, 41–42, 56
  anti-epileptic drugs (AEDs), 46
  celiac disease, 48
  corticosteroids, 44–45, 56–57, 66–67
  diet, 42–43
  diseases, 47–50
  early diagnosis, importance of, 14
  family history, 35–36, 37
  gender, 34
  hormone levels, low, 56
  inflammatory bowel disease, 47
  lifestyle factors, 40–43
  list of, 14
  medications, 43–47
  menstrual periods, starting and stopping age, 40
  reducing risks, 50–51
  smoking, 40–41, 56
  stomach surgery, 48
  thyroid medication excess, 45
  weight, 36–40
Rubin, Alan L., MD (*Thyroid For Dummies*), 45
Ryan, Tony (*Cross-Training For Dummies*), 104

• S •

salt
  dietary intake, 82
  effect on calcium, 43, 82
sarcoidosis, 175
Scheuermann's disease (juvenile epiphysitis), 116
Schlosberg, Suzanne (*Weight Training For Dummies*), 104, 240
scoliosis
  height loss, 116, 246
  idiopathic juvenile osteoporosis (IJO), 65
  osteogenesis imperfecta (OI), 65
  osteoporosis and, 246
SD (standard deviation), 140, 268
seeds, as calcium source, 75, 228–229
seizure medications, 46
selective estrogen receptor modulators (SERMs), 268
sesmoid bones, 21
shopping wisely, 248
short bones, 22
Single Energy X-Ray Absorptiometry (SXA), 137
skin cancer, 163
smoking
  effect on bone density, 15, 233
  effect on fracture frequency, 56
  helping teens to avoid, 250
  osteoporosis and, 40–41
sodas, 43
sodium
  intake, 82
  storage in bone, 234
South Carolina, osteoporosis program, 259–260
South Dakota, osteoporosis program, 260
soymilk
  children and, 248–249
  for lactose intolerant patients, 77
spinal compression fractures. *See* vertebral compression fractures
spongy bone, 268. *See also* trabecular bone
sprue. *See* celiac disease
standard deviation (SD), 140, 268
state osteoporosis programs
  Alabama, 251
  Alaska, 251
  Arizona, 252
  Arkansas, 252
  California, 252
  Colorado, 252
  Connecticut, 253
  Delaware, 253
  District of Columbia, 253
  Florida, 253
  Georgia, 254
  Hawaii, 254
  Idaho, 254
  Illinois, 254
  Indiana, 254
  Iowa, 255
  Kansas, 255
  Kentucky, 255
  Louisiana, 255
  Maine, 255
  Maryland, 255
  Massachusetts, 256
  Michigan, 223, 256
  Minnesota, 256
  Mississippi, 256
  Missouri, 256
  Montana, 257
  Nebraska, 257
  Nevada, 257
  New Hampshire, 257
  New Jersey, 223, 257
  New Mexico, 258
  New York, 258
  North Carolina, 223, 258
  North Dakota, 258
  Ohio, 258
  Oklahoma, 258–259
  Oregon, 259
  Pennsylvania, 259
  Rhode Island, 259
  South Carolina, 259–260
  South Dakota, 260
  Tennessee, 260
  Texas, 260
  Utah, 260
  Vermont, 260
  Virginia, 260
  Washington, 261

West Virginia, 261
Wisconsin, 261
Wyoming, 261
statistics, related to osteoporosis, 11–12
steroid hormone (DHEA), 58
stockings, compression, 203
stomach surgery, bone loss after, 48
stress fracture, 113
strontium ranelate (Protelos)
definition, 268
side effects, 160
use, 159–160
sunlight, vitamin D and, 64, 80, 162–163
supplements
calcium, 167–175
vitamin A, 166–167
vitamin D, 162–166
support groups
doctor recommendations, 125
online, 239–240
resources, 239
Surgeon General
as information resource, 222
statistics from, 11, 108
Web site, 222, 242
surgery
complications, 202–203
hip, 198–206
hospitalization, 201–202
kyphoplasty, 208–209, 220–221
physical activity after, 203–204
physical therapy after, 204–205
planning for, 199–200
revision, 206
for vertebral compression fractures, 208–209, 220–221
swimming, 90, 188, 203
SXA (Single Energy X-Ray Absorptiometry), 137
synthetic estrogen (Estren), 219

• T •

tacos, as calcium source, 229
T'ai Chi For Dummies (Therese Iknoian and Manny Fuentes), 210
tanning salon, 163
tannins, 171
teenager
anorexia nervosa, 6–61
bulimia, 61–62
dieting and bone loss, 60–62
female athlete triad, 62–63
Tennessee, osteoporosis program, 260
TENS (Transcutaneous Electrical Nerve Stimulation) unit, 189
teriparatide (rhPTH) (Forteo), 268
teripeptide, 156
testosterone
andropause and, 56
chemotherapy effect on, 56, 59
contraindications for use, 157–158
definition, 268
drugs that lower, 46
forms of medication, 157
function of, 28
side effects, 157
treatment with, 58
tetracycline, 171
Texas, osteoporosis program, 260
therapy, evaluating, 16
thoracic spine, 116
Thoracic-Lumbar-Sacral Orthosis (TLSO), 208
thromboembolic disease, 154
Thyroid For Dummies (Alan L. Rubin, MD), 45
thyroid gland
calcitonin production, 27
definition, 268
overactive, 50
thyroid medication, 171
tibolone (Livial), 160, 269
TLSO (Thoracic-Lumbar-Sacral Orthosis), 208
total hip replacement, 198. *See also* hip replacement
trabecular bone
definition, 22, 269
healing time, 212
location, 22–23
loss of, 23
remodeling and, 24
Transcutaneous Electrical Nerve Stimulation (TENS) unit, 189

trapezius muscle, 98
treatment. *See also* medications; pain management; surgery
  plan setup, 124–125
  T-score and bisphosphonate treatment decision, 148–149
tribasic calcium phosphate, 168–169
triceps kickback (exercise), 96–97
T-score
  bisphosphonate treatment decision and, 148–149
  definition, 268
  meaning of, 140–141
  World Health Organization definitions and, 141
Tylenol (acetaminophen), 17, 182

• U •

ulcerative colitis, 47
ulna, 110
Ultra Lactaid tablets, 77
ultrasound
  for bone density testing, 139
  definition, 269
ultraviolet light, 162–163
urine tests, of bone turnover, 139
U.S. Department of Health and Human Services, 41
Utah, osteoporosis program, 260
uterine cancer, 150, 151

• V •

vegetables, as calcium source, 78, 228
veins, blood clots in, 154
Vermont, osteoporosis program, 260
vertebrae, definition, 269
vertebral compression fractures
  burst, 207, 264
  complications, 207
  consequences of, 114–117
  description, 114–117, 269
  diagnosis, 207
  dowager's hump caused by, 114, 115, 220
  frequency of, 12
  height loss, 11, 36
  location of, 208
  pain from, 115, 116, 179
  recovering from, 209–210
  statistics, 117, 197, 206
  treatment, 208–209, 220–221
  wedge, 114, 115, 207, 269
vertebroplasty
  definition, 269
  kyphoplasty compared, 209, 220, 221
  percutaneous vertebroplasty procedure, 190, 208
Viactiv, 172, 174
videos, 240
Vioxx, 183, 184
Virginia, osteoporosis program, 260
vitamin A, effect on bone resorption, 46, 166–167
vitamin D
  alcohol effect on, 42
  amount in multivitamin supplements, 164
  blood levels, checking, 164
  combined with calcium, 173
  daily requirement, 50, 56, 217
  deficiency and rickets, 63–64
  deficiency from gastrointestinal diseases, 47–48
  definition, 269
  drugs interfering with absorption of, 64, 164
  effect of anti-epileptic drugs on, 46
  falls, reduction with vitamin D supplementation, 165
  food sources of, 80
  functions of, 27, 162
  hip fractures and vitamin D deficiency, 165
  recommended daily intake, 163
  renal osteodystrophy and, 49
  research on, 216–217
  role of, 80

sources of, 162
sunlight and, 64, 80, 162–163
toxicity, 165–166
vitamin K, 174
vitamin supplements, amount of ingredients in, 162
vitamind.ucr.edu (Web site), 242
volumetric CT scanning, 217

• W •

walkers, 199–200, 205, 209
warfarin (Coumadin), 174, 184, 203
Washington, osteoporosis program, 261
Web sites
American College of Rheumatology, 185, 214, 242
American Society for Bone and Mineral Research (ASBMR), 214
back.com, 208
Bone and Joint Decade project, 221
Eli Lilly, 242
Got Milk?, 74
Harvard Medical School, 239
hiprotector.com, 196
International Osteoporosis Foundation (IOF), 222
Kaiser Family Foundation, 130
Livial, 160
Mayo Clinic, 239
Medicare, 129
medlineplus.com, 242
medscape.com, 242
Merck, 242
National Institute on Aging, 104, 240
National Institute on Aging Information Center (NIAIC), 238
National Institutes of Health (NIH), 222
National Osteoporosis Foundation (NOF), 214, 237–238
NIH Osteoporosis and Related Bone Diseases-National Resource Center, 238
osteo.org, 238
Procter & Gamble, 242
rheumatology.org, 17, 242
state osteoporosis programs, 251–261
Surgeon General's office, 222
vitamind.ucr.edu, 242
whymilk.com, 242
World Health Organization (WHO), 221
wedge fracture
creation of, 114
definition, 207, 269
dowager's hump and, 115
weight
body mass index (BMI), 37–39
effect on bones, 85–86
as risk factor for osteoporosis, 36–37, 40
weight training. *See* resistance training
Weight Training For Dummies (Liz Neporent and Suzanne Schlosberg), 104, 240
weight-bearing exercise, 89–90, 244, 269
West Virginia, osteoporosis program, 261
whymilk.com (Web site), 242
Wisconsin, osteoporosis program, 261
women's Health Initiative Memory study, 151
World Health Organization (WHO)
Bone and Joint Decade project, 221
T-scores and osteoporosis definitions, 141
Web site, 221
World Osteoporosis Day, 222
wormian bones, 21
wrist fractures
description, 109–110
diagnosis, 210
frequency of, 12
statistics on, 197
treatment, 210
Wyoming, osteoporosis program, 261

• X •

X-ray, 134, 198, 207, 210, 245. *See also* Dual Energy X-Ray Absorptiometry (DXA)

• Y •

yogurt, 75, 77
Yorkey, Mike (*Fitness Over Forty For Dummies*), 240

• Z •

zoledronic acid (Zometa)
  definition, 269
  dosage, 219
  intravenous, 158–159
  study on, 159
  use in bone cancer, 158
Z-score
  definition, 269
  interpretation of, 141–142

SPORTS, FITNESS, PARENTING, RELIGION & SPIRITUALITY

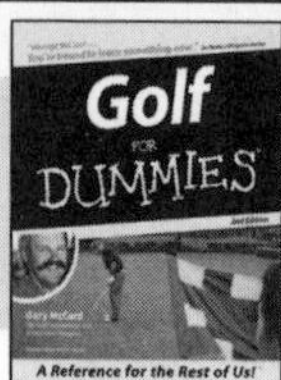

0-7645-5146-9

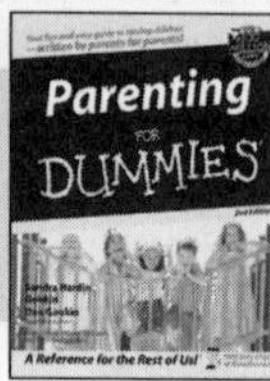

0-7645-5418-2

Also available:

- Adoption For Dummies 0-7645-5488-3
- Basketball For Dummies 0-7645-5248-1
- The Bible For Dummies 0-7645-5296-1
- Buddhism For Dummies 0-7645-5359-3
- Catholicism For Dummies 0-7645-5391-7
- Hockey For Dummies 0-7645-5228-7
- Judaism For Dummies 0-7645-5299-6
- Martial Arts For Dummies 0-7645-5358-5
- Pilates For Dummies 0-7645-5397-6
- Religion For Dummies 0-7645-5264-3
- Teaching Kids to Read For Dummies 0-7645-4043-2
- Weight Training For Dummies 0-7645-5168-X
- Yoga For Dummies 0-7645-5117-5

TRAVEL

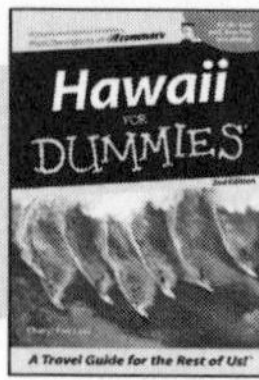

0-7645-5438-7

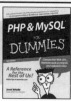

0-7645-5453-0

Also available:

- Alaska For Dummies 0-7645-1761-9
- Arizona For Dummies 0-7645-6938-4
- Cancún and the Yucatán For Dummies 0-7645-2437-2
- Cruise Vacations For Dummies 0-7645-6941-4
- Europe For Dummies 0-7645-5456-5
- Ireland For Dummies 0-7645-5455-7
- Las Vegas For Dummies 0-7645-5448-4
- London For Dummies 0-7645-4277-X
- New York City For Dummies 0-7645-6945-7
- Paris For Dummies 0-7645-5494-8
- RV Vacations For Dummies 0-7645-5443-3
- Walt Disney World & Orlando For Dummies 0-7645-6943-0

GRAPHICS, DESIGN & WEB DEVELOPMENT

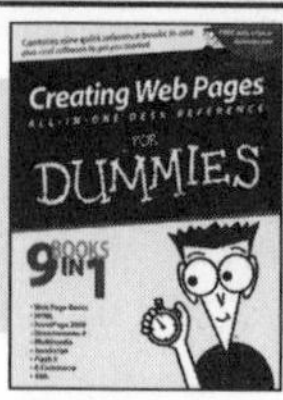

0-7645-4345-8

0-7645-5589-8

Also available:

- Adobe Acrobat 6 PDF For Dummies 0-7645-3760-1
- Building a Web Site For Dummies 0-7645-7144-3
- Dreamweaver MX 2004 For Dummies 0-7645-4342-3
- FrontPage 2003 For Dummies 0-7645-3882-9
- HTML 4 For Dummies 0-7645-1995-6
- Illustrator CS For Dummies 0-7645-4084-X
- Macromedia Flash MX 2004 For Dummies 0-7645-4358-X
- Photoshop 7 All-in-One Desk Reference For Dummies 0-7645-1667-1
- Photoshop CS Timesaving Techniques For Dummies 0-7645-6782-9
- PHP 5 For Dummies 0-7645-4166-8
- PowerPoint 2003 For Dummies 0-7645-3908-6
- QuarkXPress 6 For Dummies 0-7645-2593-X

NETWORKING, SECURITY, PROGRAMMING & DATABASES

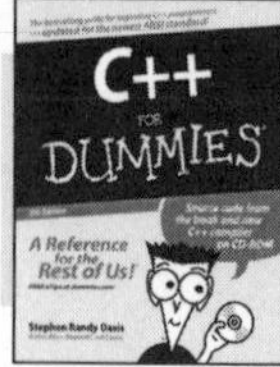

0-7645-6852-3

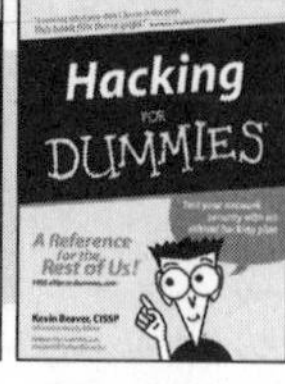

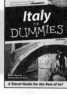

0-7645-5784-X

Also available:

- A+ Certification For Dummies 0-7645-4187-0
- Access 2003 All-in-One Desk Reference For Dummies 0-7645-3988-4
- Beginning Programming For Dummies 0-7645-4997-9
- C For Dummies 0-7645-7068-4
- Firewalls For Dummies 0-7645-4048-3
- Home Networking For Dummies 0-7645-42796
- Network Security For Dummies 0-7645-1679-5
- Networking For Dummies 0-7645-1677-9
- TCP/IP For Dummies 0-7645-1760-0
- VBA For Dummies 0-7645-3989-2
- Wireless All In-One Desk Reference For Dummies 0-7645-7496-5
- Wireless Home Networking For Dummies 0-7645-3910-8

HEALTH & SELF-HELP

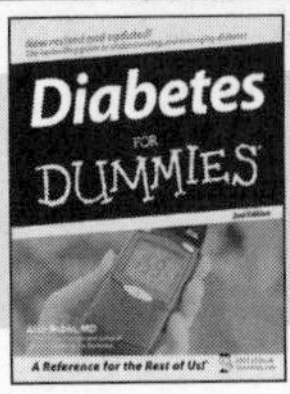

0-7645-6820-5 *†

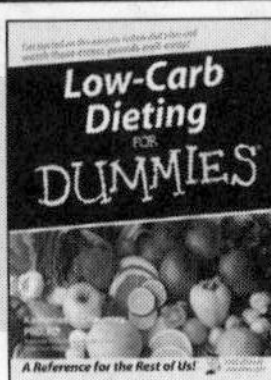

0-7645-2566-2

Also available:

- Alzheimer's For Dummies 0-7645-3899-3
- Asthma For Dummies 0-7645-4233-8
- Controlling Cholesterol For Dummies 0-7645-5440-9
- Depression For Dummies 0-7645-3900-0
- Dieting For Dummies 0-7645-4149-8
- Fertility For Dummies 0-7645-2549-2
- Fibromyalgia For Dummies 0-7645-5441-7
- Improving Your Memory For Dummies 0-7645-5435-2
- Pregnancy For Dummies † 0-7645-4483-7
- Quitting Smoking For Dummies 0-7645-2629-4
- Relationships For Dummies 0-7645-5384-4
- Thyroid For Dummies 0-7645-5385-2

EDUCATION, HISTORY, REFERENCE & TEST PREPARATION

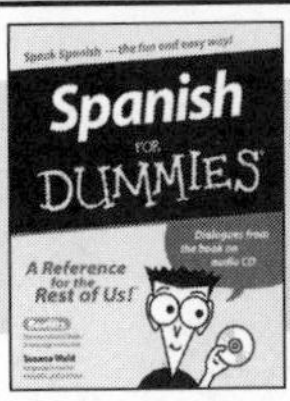

0-7645-5194-9

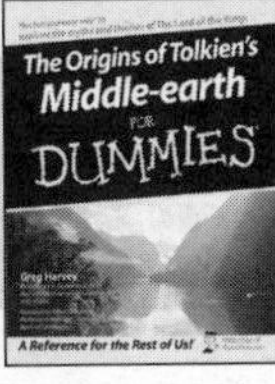

0-7645-4186-2

Also available:

- Algebra For Dummies 0-7645-5325-9
- British History For Dummies 0-7645-7021-8
- Calculus For Dummies 0-7645-2498-4
- English Grammar For Dummies 0-7645-5322-4
- Forensics For Dummies 0-7645-5580-4
- The GMAT For Dummies 0-7645-5251-1
- Inglés Para Dummies 0-7645-5427-1
- Italian For Dummies 0-7645-5196-5
- Latin For Dummies 0-7645-5431-X
- Lewis & Clark For Dummies 0-7645-2545-X
- Research Papers For Dummies 0-7645-5426-3
- The SAT I For Dummies 0-7645-7193-1
- Science Fair Projects For Dummies 0-7645-5460-3
- U.S. History For Dummies 0-7645-5249-X

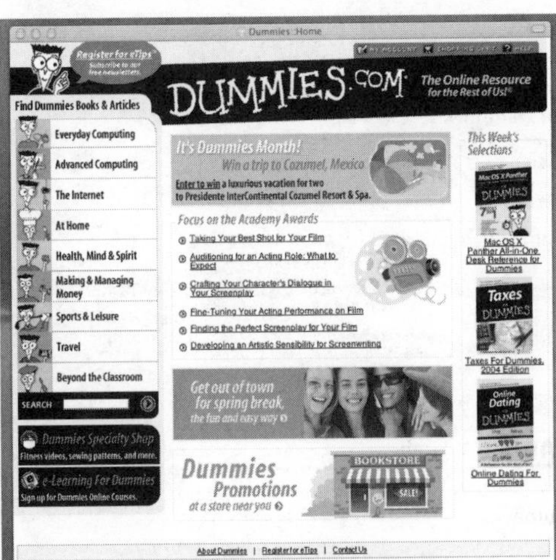

Get smart @ dummies.com®

- **Find a full list of Dummies titles**
- **Look into loads of FREE on-site articles**
- **Sign up for FREE eTips e-mailed to you weekly**
- **See what other products carry the Dummies name**
- **Shop directly from the Dummies bookstore**
- **Enter to win new prizes every month!**

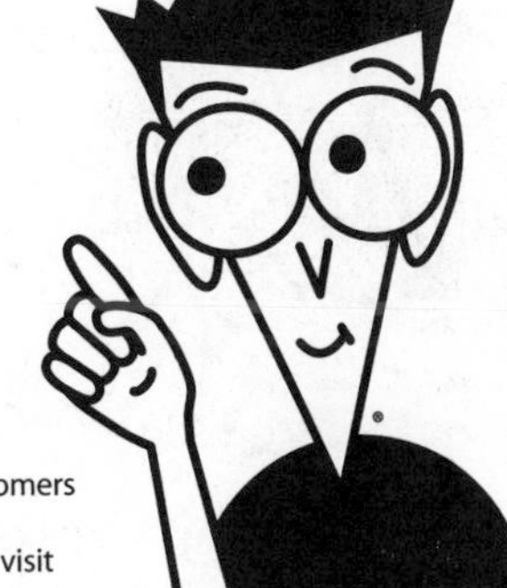

*** Separate Canadian edition also available**
† Separate U.K. edition also available

Available wherever books are sold. For more information or to order direct: U.S. customers visit www.dummies.com or call 1-877-762-2974.
U.K. customers visit www.wileyeurope.com or call 0800 243407. Canadian customers visit www.wiley.ca or call 1-800-567-4797.

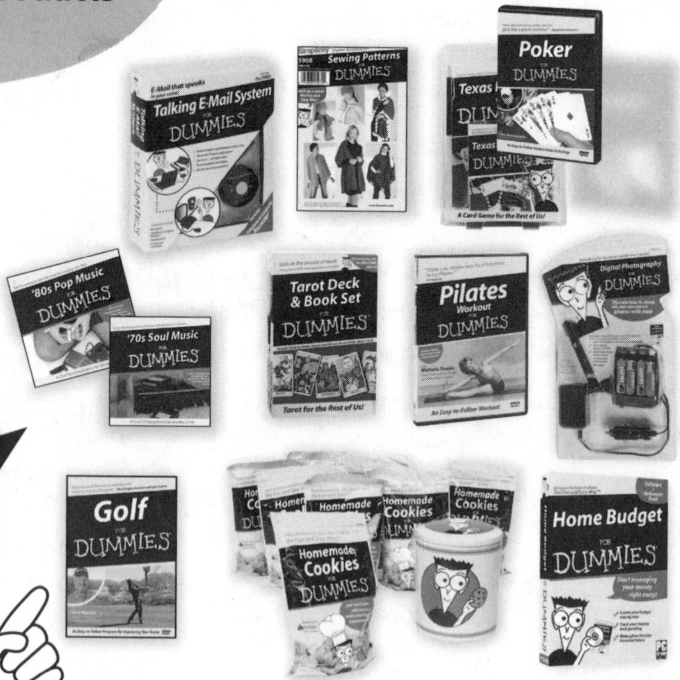

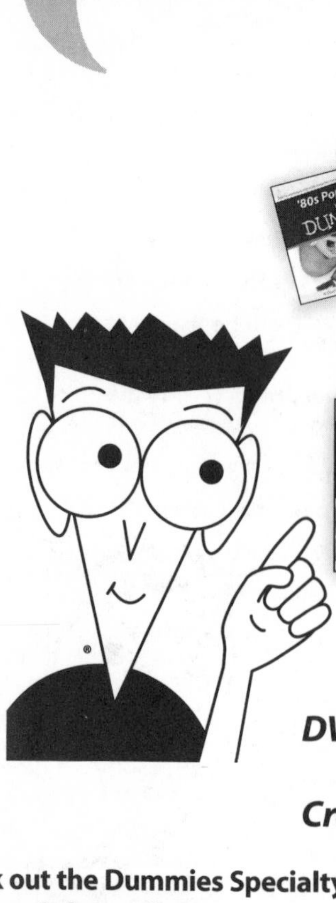